THE BENEFICIAL EFFECTS OF THIS POWERFUL PHYTONUTRIENT

Resveratrol, a natural product derived from grapes, has potent antioxidant properties that make it effective against damaging free radicals. This guide explains the nutritional and therapeutic effects of red wine, often associated with a decrease in heart disease in moderate drinkers. Resveratrol's other beneficial health effects include acting as an anti-inflammatory, promoting anticancer activities, and reducing the risk of blood clots and high blood pressure.

ABOUT THE AUTHOR

Dr. Bagchi received his Ph.D. degree in Medicinal Chemistry in 1982. He conducted post-doctoral research on free radicals and antioxidants at the University of Connecticut School of Medicine, Farmington, Connecticut. Presently, he is an Associate Professor in the Department of Pharmaceutical and Administrative Sciences at the Creighton University School of Pharmacy and Allied Health Professions in Omaha, Nebraska. His research interests include free radicals, human diseases, and the protective role of antioxidants. Dr. Bagchi is actively engaged in assessing the intricate issues of cell death and the mechanistic pathways of antioxidant cytoprotection. Dr. Bagchi and coworkers have published more than a hundred papers on free radicals and antioxidants in peer-reviewed journals. He has delivered invited lectures at various national and international conferences. Dr. Bagchi is a Fellow of the American College of Nutrition, a member of the Society of Toxicology, the New York Academy of Sciences, and the TCE [trichloroethylene] stakeholder Committee of the Wright-Patterson Air Force Base in Ohio. He has been inducted into the Phi Beta Delta Honor Society for International Scholars. Recently, Dr. Bagchi was appointed as a Member of the Study Section and Peer Review Committee of the National Institutes of Health.

Dr. Bagchi's research projects are funded by the U.S. Air Force Office of Scientific Research, the Nebraska State Department of Health, a Biomedical Research Support Grant from NIH, the National Cancer Institute (NIH), Health Future Foundation, The Procter & Gamble Company, and Abbott Laboratories.

Resveratrol and Human Health

Debasis Bagchi, Ph.D., F.A.C.N.

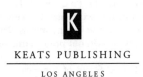

KEATS PUBLISHING

LOS ANGELES

NTC/Contemporary Publishing Group

Resveratrol and Human Health is intended solely for informational and educational purposes and not as medical advice. Please consult a medical or health professional if you have questions about your health.

RESVERATROL AND HUMAN HEALTH

Published by Keats Publishing
A division of NTC/Contemporary Publishing Group, Inc.
4255 West Touhy Avenue, Lincolnwood, Illinois 60712, U.S.A.

Printed and bound in the United States of America
International Standard Book Number: 0-87983-955-4
00 01 02 03 04 RCP 18 17 16 15 14 13 12 11 10 9 8 7 6 5 4 3 2 1

Contents

In recent years, a newfound interest has surfaced in the health benefits of drinking moderate amounts of wine. Evidence from many epidemiological studies involving thousands of human subjects supports the notion that moderate wine consumption lowers the risk for cardiovascular heart disease and death. Approximately half of this risk reduction may be attributed to increased concentrations of circulating high-density lipoprotein cholesterol (also known as HDL-C or the good cholesterol), which are increased by wine in a dose-dependent manner. Lipoproteins are proteins that transport fats (lipids) to various tissues. They are necessary for the proper function of many biological systems, but too much LDL, or too little HDL, can result in an increased risk for heart disease. There are many other risk factors for heart disease, and it is now known that cholesterol plays a smaller role than previously thought, but high LDL is still regarded as a risk factor for atherosclerosis. Reduced platelet coagulability is another mechanism that is thought to play a beneficial role in this process. This means that the tendency to have blood clots is reduced.

However, other mechanisms such as inhibition of lipoprotein oxidation, free-radical scavenging, and modulation of eicosanoid metabolism may reduce the likelihood of atherosclerosis and its sequelae, including coronary heart disease, in moderate wine drinkers. Lipoprotein oxidation means that detrimental biochemical reactions involving free radicals can react with lipoproteins, even if they are at normal levels. This reaction can cause the events that lead to the deposition of fats and cholesterol in the arteries. This theory helps to explain why a majority of people who have heart disease often have normal cholesterol levels. Because of its chemistry, alcohol (ethanol) in wine is unlikely to account for all of the antioxidant effects; a great deal of interest is being focused on finding a suitable explanation.[1]

Resveratrol, a nonalcoholic constituent of wine, has been identified with a broad spectrum of health benefits. Resveratrol (3, 5, 4'-trihydroxystilbene) is a naturally occurring phenolic antioxidant compound abundant in grapes, peanuts, lilly, pine, and other plants. Phenolic is a chemical word that places resveratrol into a specific chemical group of compounds. These will be discussed later in this Good Health Guide. Resveratrol is classified as a natural plant antibiotic known as *phytoalexin*, which confers disease resistance in the plant kingdom, and is produced under adverse conditions such as environmental stress, fungal infection, and pathogenic (bacterial) attack. Structurally, resveratrol is a *stilbene,* the parent skeleton structure of a family of compounds including the *cis-* and *trans*-isomers; glucosides of *cis-* and *trans*-isomers *cis*-polydatin and *trans*-polydatin; dimers (ε-viniferin), trimers (α–viniferin), and tetramers (γ-viniferin) of resveratrol; and other resveratrol polymers. The *trans* form of the resveratrol molecule is virtually the only naturally occurring form, as is true with most molecules in nature.

Resveratrol has long been used as an important component of an Ayurvedic medicine called Darakchasava and a Chinese medicine called *Ko-jo-kon,* which is claimed to have protective effects against arteriosclerosis, coronary heart diseases, women's postmenopausal problems, and a broad spectrum of degenerative diseases. The roots of some plants (especially *Polygonum cuspidatum*, a traditional Chinese herb also known as *Hu-Chang*) that contain resveratrol have been used to treat diseases such as hyperlipidemia (too much fat in the blood), arteriosclerosis, allergic diseases, and various inflammatory diseases.

According to the Oriental *Materia Medica*, traditional uses of *Polygonum cuspidatum* root are to clear up "heat," invigorate blood, detoxify, and reduce swelling. Oriental cultures have used this root for centuries to treat dysentery, headache, amenorrhea, mastitis, external trauma, inflammatory and allergic diseases, hyperlipidemia, and arteriosclerosis. In Chinese medicine, *Polygonum cuspidatum* root is used to treat bacterial and viral infections, scalds and burns, cough, asthma, arthritis, hepatitis, inflammatory diseases, hypertension, and cancer.

Some studies suggest that resveratrol protects against low-density lipoprotein (LDL) oxidation and promotes many biological attributes that favor cardioprotection, vascular relaxation, antioxidant activity, modulation of hepatic (liver) lipid synthesis, and inhibition of platelet aggregation, as well as inhibition of pro-atherogenic eicosanoids derived from fatty acids. Eicosanoids are hormones—the molecules that regulate almost everything that happens in our body, and the messengers of the body that send signals to various cells and tissues. Resveratrol also possesses the ability to prevent liver injury induced by administration of peroxidized oil. Furthermore, it has been reported that stilbenes showed antileukemic activity due to their effect on arachidonate metabolism in leukocytes[2]. Arachidonate is the polyunsaturated fatty acid that is the precursor of the eicosanoid hormones mentioned above.

In a recent study published in the journal *Science*, resveratrol was found to act as an antimutagen and potent chemopreventive (cancer preventive) agent by inhibiting the cellular events associated with cancer initiation, promotion, and progression.[3] These three factors are generally accepted as important mechanistic steps in cancer development. Among the many attributes of resveratrol named by this study, the most exciting are as follows:

- induced Phase II–drug-metabolizing enzymes (anti-initiation activity)

- mediated anti-inflammatory effects and inhibited cyclooxygenase (COX) and hydroperoxidase functions (antipromotion activity)
- induced human promyelocytic leukemia cell differentiation (anti-progression activity)
- inhibited the development of preneoplastic lesions in carcinogen-treated mouse mammary glands in culture and inhibited tumorigenesis in a mouse skin cancer model.

What all this means is that many cellular processes that are known to contribute to cancer were changed by resveratrol such that the risk of cancer was reduced.

Another recent study indicates that resveratrol directly stimulates cell proliferation and differentiation of osteoblasts. Differentiation is a very important aspect of our cells that is related to cancer. Our cells, under normal development, differentiate to become specific types of cells. We have skin cells, liver cells, heart muscle cells, etc. All of these differentiated cells work together to maintain the function of an organ or tissue. Cancer cells are not differentiated, and if our cells change to become cancerous they are considered *dedifferentiated*. This means that they no longer work together, but actually multiply uncontrollably. There is no cellular communication that tells the cells to stop multiplying and to work together. Therefore, any substance or nutritional component that keeps cells differentiated represents a way to minimize cancer cell formation.

Resveratrol has been shown to decrease tumor growth *in vivo* (in a living being) Despite the information that we already have, there is still much we do not know about the effects of resveratrol and the other polyphenolic constituents in wine. There is ongoing debate about the exact mechanism of action by which the desired effects of resveratrol take place. Is resveratrol even the best stilbene? Many questions remain, but preliminary results look very promising. Among the many attributes of resveratrol named by these studies, its most exciting properties are the following:

- a potent free-radical scavenger
- an anti-inflammatory agent

- promotes antimutagenic, antitumor, and anticancer activities
- a novel cardioprotectant
- protects against LDL oxidation and protects against chronic ischemia[4]
- reduces myocardial infarction and ischemia-reperfusion injury
- promotes vascular relaxation through the generation of nitric oxide[5]
- a potent antiperoxidant and inhibitor of lysosomal enzymes
- a protein-tyrosine kinase inhibitor
- a powerful inhibitor of human platelet aggregation and serotonin secretion
- a novel phytoestrogen: a safe natural replacement for estrogen during menopause
- a novel neuroprotectant
- ameliorates depression
- increases collagen synthesis
- reduces the risk of osteoporosis and increases bone formation
- helps balance mood swings

These properties are very exciting because they represent many of the known risks for developing different degenerative diseases. It is important to understand that there are many other risk factors associated with disease and that the consumption of resveratrol may be one of many important steps in risk reduction.

THE FRENCH PARADOX AND CORONARY HEART DISEASE

A resurgence of interest has recently been focused on the roles of wine, and therefore resveratrol, in the diet based on the phenomenon called "the French paradox." Early epidemiological studies indicated that in most developed countries, high dietary intakes of saturated fat, cholesterol, total fat, and total caloric intake correlate positively with mortality from heart disease. However, more recent and larger studies suggest the high-fat theory is not a major factor in heart disease. Epidemiological studies are difficult to interpret and they can sometimes be used as proof of an idea, when, in fact, all that can be obtained from them is a trend, but never direct proof.

However, St. Leger and his colleagues[1] conducted an epidemiological study in 1979 that demonstrated a significant reduction in mortality from coronary heart disease with higher consumption of wine. French people are known to consume foods high in saturated fats and cholesterol, yet they have a low mortality rate from coronary heart disease.[2,3] The discovery that the saturated fat intake in France is similar to that of other developed countries, while French mortality from coronary heart disease is only one-third the average of such countries, has become known as the French paradox.[2-4] There are probably other important environmental factors that contribute to this paradox, such as total calorie intake, exercise, or sugar intake, but wine consumption was the basis of this study.

The major risk factors of coronary heart diseases are high levels of LDL (low-density lipoprotein) in blood, hypertension (high blood pressure), obesity, smoking, and a sedentary lifestyle.[5,6] The main causes of death from coronary heart disease are myocardial infarction (heart attack), increased thrombogenic activity (blood clots), and atherosclerosis.[5,6]

Coronary heart disease may be defined as "atherosclerosis of the coronary arteries." Atherosclerosis causes cerebrovascular and cardiovascular disease, leading to ischemic stroke and myocardial infarction, respectively, and causes more than 40 percent of all deaths in Western civilization.[1-3] Atherosclerosis is a disease that results in abnormally thickened regions of the vascular wall. These regions, called plaques, are characterized by atypical proliferations of modified smooth muscle cells and deposits of large quantities of cholesterol in the form of "foam cells" just beneath the endothelium. As plaque development narrows arteries, decreased blood supply may cause damage to the heart or brain. Because the plaque is an abnormal surface, a clot may form on it and eventually block the artery, causing either a heart attack or stroke. A clot is a web of threadlike fibrin molecules that forms a patch over the break in the blood vessel. Clots are dissolved naturally by plasmin, an enzyme formed from the plasma protein plasminogen. Tissue type plasminogen activator is capable of converting plasmin to plasminogen.[5,6]

Arteriosclerosis is another type of mechanism that leads to narrowing of the arteries, but in this case the arteries become brittle and they are narrowed by calcification, without the presence of significant amounts of fats and cholesterol. It is important to note that it has been known for many years that more people die of heart disease who have normal levels of cholesterol than do those who have high levels of cholesterol. This fact suggests that protection from wine, and therefore from resveratrol, is more important in reducing the oxidation of cholesterol than in reducing its amount in the blood.

The French paradox seems to confirm this. In France there is a contrast between foods rich in saturated fat and cholesterol, and a lower mortality rate from coronary heart disease, that is observed in Mediterranean countries where the dietary fat intake is much lower compared to France. The French have a high intake of saturated fat (14 to 15 percent of energy), which is similar to amounts consumed in the United Kingdom and the United States. In the U.K. and the U.S.,[7] this diet has been thought to lead to high serum cholesterol concentrations and elevated rates of coronary heart disease. However, mortality rates from coronary heart disease in France are much closer to those in the Mediterranean countries, Japan, and China, where such rates are less than one-third of that in North America.[7,8] Lifestyle appears to play a role in the French paradox: France was reported to have the highest wine intake and the highest total alcohol intake with the second lowest mortality rate from coronary heart disease in the world.[2] This finding suggests a protective effect of wine no matter how much fat is consumed.

Studies have shown that consumption of wine at levels seen in France (20 to 30 gms per day) can reduce the risk of coronary heart disease by at least 40 percent.[2,3,7] A study conducted in Denmark between 1976 and 1988, involving 13,285 human subjects, demonstrated that a low to moderate intake of wine was associated with lower mortality from cardiovascular and cerebrovascular disease, while a similar intake of spirits (hard liquor) implied an increased risk.[4,7–9] The protective effect of red wine was observed in men and women, in the elderly, and in smokers and nonsmokers. Thus, moderate consumption of wine has been seen to lower the risk for development of atherosclerosis and coronary artery disease. This has been especially true in France and other Mediterranean areas where wine is an integral part of the diet.[7–10]

Because a distinguishing feature of the French diet is the regular consumption of red wine with meals, epidemiological studies have focused on the correlation between wine consumption and the reduced risk of coronary heart disease.[9] Several wine components show promise for their possible cardiovascular protective effects,[5] including the alcohol itself, polyphenolic components such as bioflavonoids and proanthocyanidins, and components of grape skin, such as resveratrol and nitric oxide. Polyphenolic constituents including bioflavonoids, proanthocyanidins, and resveratrol can function as potential antioxidants or decrease the incidence of thrombosis. Nitric oxide has been found to relax aortic endothelium, and lower nitric oxide levels may lead to hyperlipidemia in rats.[11,12] The ability of wine to demonstrate such beneficial effects was attributed to its high content of polyphenolic constituents such as bioflavonoids, proanthocyanidins, and resveratrol. The cardioprotective ability of alcohol may be due to its effect on the fibrinolytic factors or due to the high-density lipoprotein concentrations.[10,11] However, caution is required when making recommendations for daily alcohol consumption, as several researchers have reported a negative association between alcohol consumption and cardiovascular disease.

HISTORY OF WINE

The term "wine" refers to the fermented juice of the grape. Grapes naturally contain the vital ingredients for fermentation because they are rich in sugar and have a waxy skin that collects wild airborne yeasts. Sometimes other fruit juices are used to prepare wine, and the name of the fruit usually precedes the word "wine." In literature, wine has been demonstrated as one of the oldest medicines in the world, and has been used as a base for many tonics.

Historians believe that primitive peoples of the Eurasian continent may have enjoyed fermented juices from spoiled wild fruit long before grapes were first cultivated, some 7,000 years ago in the region around the Caspian Sea. Archaeologists have found pottery wine jars 6,000 to 7,000 years old, suggesting that the first wines were made in the Middle East from grapes, figs, and dates. The art of grape cultivation spread westward with migratory people, especially the Jews—the Bible mentions that Noah raised grapes and made wine. Egyptian accounts of winemaking date back to about 2500 B.C. Egyptians also stored jars of wine in special wine cellars dug out of the earth; they must have realized that wine is best preserved when stored in a cool environment. The ancient Greek, Minoan, and Etruscan civilizations also produced wine for their own use, as well as for trading, as evidenced by the airtight clay jars they used as containers. The Greeks organized symposiums at which people gathered for intellectual discussions, with wine drinking as an integral part of the event.

The Romans were the first to retard the spoilage of wine by storing wine in their smokehouses. They also became experts in growing vines and vineyards, and helped to spread vine-growing techniques throughout their European colonies. Roman wine festivals (also known as Bacchanalia, after the Roman God of wine, Bacchus) were characterized by participants drinking to intoxication, and so resembled the Dionysian orgies. Notably, the Romans did not allow women to drink wine. By the early Christian era, the Gauls in France rivaled the Romans in their wine-making skills. When the Roman Empire fell, each region of Europe made its own types of wines from the grapes of the vineyards originally cultivated by the Romans. Wine also was used sacramentally in the celebration of the Mass, with monasteries developing special recipes for making local wines. Some groups of monks, especially the Benedictines, also developed special distilled liquors from wine.

The European colonists of North America found fields of wild grapes when they arrived, and Vikings who landed in eastern Canada found grapes there, as well. However, the first wines made from the native American species (*Vitis labrusca*) were inferior to those made from European, or Old World, grapes (*Vitis vinifera*). In 1769, these European or Old World varieties were successfully cultivated and introduced into California by the Spanish priest Father Junípero Serra, who founded a string of missions with vineyards. By the nineteenth century, many European varieties of wine grapes were brought to North America—mostly to the western United States, where the vines grew well in the mild climate. Better native American grapes were developed after 1852, when the Concord grape was first grown by E. W. Bull of Concord, Massachusetts.

The growth of the American wine industry was partially

interrupted between 1919 and 1933, due to Prohibition. However, both wine production and wine consumption have increased steadily ever since. Based on extensive research into viticulture and oenology, there have been many significant innovations and improvements in the production of wines. The processing steps in wine manufacturing include fermentation, clarification, and aging.

NUTRITIONAL AND THERAPEUTIC BENEFITS OF WINE

Several medicinal and therapeutic properties have been attributed to wine since being used medicinally from the time of the ancient Greek physician, Hippocrates (460 to 370 B.C.). For example, the aroma and taste of good wines are known to stimulate the appetite. The nonalcoholic constituents of wine have been demonstrated to slow the alcohol absorption rate.[1-3] Wine constituents have a relaxing effect, and also have been found to promote better absorption and utilization of the essential minerals calcium, phosphorous, magnesium and zinc, as compared to pure alcohol or water.[1,2,4] Various nutrition-related groups recommend that people consume five to seven servings of fresh fruits and vegetables daily. If followed, this could assure consumption of a healthy quantity of bioflavonoids. But if too much fruit is consumed, the sugar levels in the diet can become too high.[5] Waterhouse and Frankel[6] have estimated that the bioflavonoid content of the average North American diet could be enhanced 40 percent by consumption of two glasses of red wine per day. Red wine contains a low amount of residual sugar, so this would be a convenient way to increase bioflavanoid levels without all the sugar. In a recent review, it was postulated that if every adult in North America consumed two glasses of red wine daily, deaths from cardiovascular disease would be cut by 40 percent. Furthermore, the polyphenolic antioxidants of wine, including resveratrol, proanthocyanidins, and bioflavonoids, are known to enhance antioxidant activity, induce cancer chemoprevention, stimulate digestive functions, inhibit the peroxidation of low-density lipoprotein cholesterol (LDL-C, the so-called bad cholesterol), and reduce thrombotic tendency.[7]

A few researchers have demonstrated that red wines may induce migraine headaches or produce mutagenic, carcinogenic, and genotoxic properties at high levels. However, intoxication and adverse effects are less likely to occur when low to moderate amounts of wine are consumed.

Because of the high concentration of resveratrol in the skin of the grape, significant amounts of resveratrol are present in wine. Dr. Kovac and his collaborators[8] reported that the catechin derivatives and proanthocyanidins accumulate principally in the lignified portion of grape clusters, especially in the seeds, making red wine a potential source. During wine fermentation, the complex polymeric and glycosidic forms of flavonoids are broken down to monomeric forms; these forms remain stable in wines containing 10 percent or more alcohol.[6–10]

The potent antioxidant activity of polyphenolics in wine may play a therapeutic role in the prevention and amelioration of disease.[11–13] In one study, the effect of moderate consumption of red wine on the antioxidant system in rat liver, kidney, and plasma was evaluated for forty-five days and six months.[12] The study showed that moderate and prolonged consumption of red wine is consistent with higher protection against oxidation. The effects of ingesting red wine and white wine on serum antioxidant activity also were examined using a chemiluminescence assay. Human subjects who consumed 300 ml of red wine had their mean serum antioxidant capacity increased by 18 percent after one hour and by 11 percent after two hours of ingestion, while

300 ml of white wine produced 4 percent and 7 percent increases after one hour and two hours of ingestion, respectively. A comparison of red wine, white wine, and various fruit juices demonstrated a higher antioxidant capacity of red wine, in addition to its ability to enhance the antioxidant capacity of serum.[11–14] Antioxidant polyphenolic constituents in wine are absorbed and remain bioactive after absorption.[15–17]

Red wine has long been considered the cardioprotective beverage of choice.[13] Epidemiological studies have demonstrated an inverse relationship between alcohol consumption and death from coronary heart disease; this relationship is independent of sex or age and is associated with a reduction in all-cause morbidity and mortality. This is primarily due to a reduced risk of coronary heart disease, which is responsible for one of every three deaths in humans.[18,19] Alcohol in small amounts has been shown to increase high-density lipoprotein cholesterol (HDL-C, the so-called good cholesterol) and to reduce platelet coagulability, which explains the cardioprotective ability of alcohol.[20] Consumption of alcohol has also been associated with a protective effect on the risk of ischemic stroke.[3,6,21,22] Antioxidants in alcoholic beverages, especially polyphenolic antioxidants in red wine, are an important contribution to the protective effect of regular alcohol use against atherosclerotic cardiovascular disease. These antioxidants also protect against oxidation of low-density lipoprotein cholesterol (LDL-C, the so-called bad cholesterol), which is seen as the basis for a relatively lower incidence of coronary heart diseases.[3,5] The higher the polyphenolic content of a beverage, the greater the antioxidative effect. A human clinical study was conducted to evaluate the biological efficacy of wine on lipids, proteins, and antioxidant activity. Wine (especially red wine) demonstrated beneficial lipidemic and antioxidant effects by reducing total cholesterol and triglycerides, and elevating high-density lipoprotein (HDL-C)/total cholesterol ratios.[9] The study's authors further demonstrated that wine increases antioxidant efficacy by lowering the levels of lipid peroxides.[9] These are fat membranes that have been oxidized, and then become harmful. A reduction in oxidation should result in decreases in the oxidized product, which was observed.

Red wine polyphenolics have been shown to inhibit platelet aggregation; likewise, inhibition of thromboxane formation and thromboxane receptor antagonism were demonstrated for the antiplatelet activity of red wine.[10] In one study, mechanically stenosed coronary arteries were used in an animal model to assess the potency of red wine for the antiplatelet activity. Acute platelet-mediated thrombus formation caused cyclic flow reductions in coronary blood flow. Intravenous administration of 1.62 milliliters of red wine or 4 milliliters of red wine per kilogram body weight intragastrically eliminated the cyclic flow reductions. A blood alcohol level of greater than 0.2 grams per deciliter has been demonstrated to inhibit platelet aggregation *in vivo*. Since the animals given red wine intravenously had a blood alcohol content of 0.28 gram per deciliter, the investigators suggested that there are platelet inhibitors in red wine, in addition to ethanol. Red wine polyphenolics act as potent platelet inhibitors and also inhibit cell-mediated oxidation of lipoproteins. Data show that white wine is not as effective as red wine.

Wine and beer also stimulate the secretion of digestive enzymes, including gastrin, gastric acid, cholecystokinin (CCK), and pancreatic enzymes, all primary regulators of digestion.[9] This stimulation is remarkable in light of the many reports that show an inhibitory effect of alcohol on pancreatic secretion. The stimulatory effects of wine on the release of gastrointestinal hormones are different from those of other alcoholic beverages such as whisky, gin, vodka, or pure ethanol. This suggests that the nonalcoholic constituents of wine are partially responsible for the stimulatory effect of gastric and pancreatic secretions in humans. Both wine and beer have a potent effect on gastrin release. Stimulation of plasma gastrin levels following administration of distilled water, pure ethanol, beer, white and red wine, and whisky has been determined in human volunteers. It was found that alcoholic beverages with low ethanol content, such as white and red wine and beer, are strong stimulants of gastric acid secretion and gastrin release in humans. Nonalcoholic constituents of wine are most likely responsible for the strong stimulatory action of both beverages on gastric acid secretion and release of gastrin. Pure ethanol in low concentrations is a mild stimulant of gastric acid secretion, whereas at higher concentrations it has a mild effect or no inhibitory effect.

Americans consume 3 to 5 glasses of wine per week and usually no more than 1.5 glasses on any given occasion. Reports consistently show that moderate consumers of alcohol, in the form of wine, beer, or spirits, reduce their risk of heart disease by 25 to 45 percent and their risk of overall mortality by about 10 percent. An even stronger body of evidence, based upon the studies of diverse populations, suggests that wine consumers may have even lower risks for coronary heart disease and death from all causes. In a study by Carlos Vicente Serrano and colleagues recently reported at a meeting of the European Congress of Cardiology in Birmingham, England, data indicate there is definitely something in wine besides alcohol, (arguably polyphenolic constituents), that helps to prevent cholesterol from accumulating in arteries.[19] This study used 30 rabbits given a special high fat diet: 10 of the rabbits had 60 percent of a key coronary artery covered with atherosclerotic plaque, while 10 others who were simultaneously fed red wine had only 38 percent of the artery covered. A final group of 10 were fed nonalcoholic red wine and had only 48 percent of the artery clogged.[19]

According to a new Danish study, individuals with high LDL (bad cholesterol) levels that put them at high risk for coronary heart disease, benefited from moderate alcohol consumption. Researchers Hans Ole Hein and colleagues found that nondrinkers whose blood contains large amounts of unhealthy LDL cholesterol were much more likely to have heart disease than alcohol consumers with similar LDL levels. Initiated in 1970 and using the latest data from an ongoing Copenhagen study of 2,974 elderly men, Hein analyzed the interplay between the use of alcohol, cholesterol concentration, and heart disease, and confirmed "an overall inverse association between alcohol intake and risk of ischemic heart disease."[23]

A very important study from the Organization for Applied Scientific Research in the Netherlands provides further evidence that consuming alcohol as part of a meal appears to be of importance in reducing heart disease risk. The researchers reported in the *British Medical Journal* that alcohol consumed with a meal may prevent blood-clotting triggered by fats in the foods consumed.[24] The authors suggested that alcohol stimulates the production of blood factors that prevent blood clot formation and help to dissolve existing clots. Drinking alcohol with dinner assures that its protective effects are strongest in the evening, when fats from the dinner meal circulate through the bloodstream and stimulate blood clot formation. This protective effect of alcohol with dinner also carries over to the next morning, which is when most heart attacks take place.

Two more studies—the Harvard Health Professional Follow-up study and the Multiple Risk Factor Intervention Trial (MRFIT) study—have shown that men who consume 1 to 2 drinks per day reduce their risk of heart attack and heart surgery by 26 percent, compared to nondrinkers.[22] When consumption is increased to 3 to 4 drinks per day, heart disease risk decreases another 14 percent, but risk for alcohol-related problems increases. A Harvard study of 120,000 nurses has found the same risk reduction in women, using a little less alcohol. Interestingly, in the MRFIT study, cholesterol and fat in the diet were not strongly associated with heart disease.[22] Perhaps this was because of the wine consumption!

We have determined that wine is a beneficial component of a heart-healthy diet, and that there are constituents in wine other than alcohol that provide most of the benefits. We can now concentrate on what these components are and what they do. The latest study by Dr. Andrew Waterhouse and colleagues[20] at the University of California (Davis) pinpoints specific phenolic compounds in wine that inhibit the harmful oxidation of LDL cholesterol. The oxidation of LDL is believed to be a key step in the formation of atherosclerotic plaque. This again probably explains why cholesterol in the blood is not a significant risk factor for heart disease. It is the potential to oxidize cholesterol that is the more important factor.

In a landmark experiment that accelerated the pace of research in this relatively new field, Waterhouse and colleague, Edwin Frankel, found that wine-based antioxidants are more effective than α-tocopherol (the commonly known form of vitamin E) in protecting LDL cholesterol from harmful oxidation. They reported in *Lancet* that resveratrol, quercetin, and epicatechin—the polyphenolic constituents in wine—were much more effective than vitamin E in preventing LDL oxidation. This experiment helped researchers confirm the theory that a combination of phenolic compounds in wine perform antioxidant functions that may protect against arteriosclerosis over a prolonged period of consumption.

Compared with other dietary sources, wine contains relatively high levels of phenolics. Wine is also a diverse source, as it includes significant amounts of all the major classes of phenolics, including the flavanols, the anthocyanins, the catechins, and the procyanidins and tannins of the catechins. While whole fruits are rich sources of these compounds, chemical analysis of juices show low levels compared to wine. Apparently, normal aerobic (in the presence of oxygen) processing degrades the phenolic compounds. Wine production, on the other hand, is largely anaerobic (minimal oxygen), and thus serves as an effective method of extracting the substantial amounts of flavonoid phenolics in both the skins and the seeds of red grapes. In white wine production, the skins and seeds are separated from the juice immediately after crushing the grapes, which explains why flavonoid levels are much lower.

The combination of epidemiological, clinical, and mechanistic studies strongly suggest that red wine polyphenolics are beneficial nutrients that can reduce heart disease mortality. However, the alcohol in wine also can cause liver damage and hepatotoxicity. In order to make sound dietary recommendations for red wine polyphenolic constituents, a broad spectrum of *in vitro, in vivo,* and human clinical studies have been conducted on resveratrol. Its dramatic beneficial effects are shown in the next several chapters.

NATURAL SOURCES OF RESVERATROL

Resveratrol is found in a variety of fruit and vegetable plants used for human consumption. The plants classified as *spermatophytes* are known to have natural stilbenes and stilbene glycosides. Glycosides are sugar-like molecules. Resveratrol, a member of the stilbene group, is present in many plants, including the berries, leaves, and canes of grapevines *Vitis vinifera* (family Vitaceae) and *Vitis labrusca.* Resveratrol also is a natural constituent of bronze- and dark-skinned muscadine grapes (*Vitis rotundifolia*).[1-3] Grapes are one of the world's largest crops, with France, Italy, and Spain accounting for approximately 40 percent of the world's grapevine acreage. It has been established that resveratrol is synthesized and located in the skin but not in the fleshy part of the berries of *Vitis vinifera* or *Vitis labrusca.*[4] In contrast, the fleshy part of muscadine berries, or grapes, have been shown to contain resveratrol, as well as berries, pomace, and seeds. Dark-skinned muscadine grapes have slightly higher concentrations of resveratrol than do the bronze-skinned grapes. It is noteworthy to mention that muscadine grapes are resistant to many insects and diseases to which *V. vinifera* grapes are susceptible.

One of the richest sources of resveratrol is the weed *Polygonum cuspidatum*, the root extract of which has been used in Asian countries to treat headache, amenorrhea, dysentery, microbial and viral infections, inflammatory and allergic responses, asthma, arthritis, hepatitis, trauma, hyperlipidemia and arteriosclerosis, hypertension, and cancer. The root extracts of *Polygonum cuspidatum*, known as *Hu-Chang* and *Ko-jo-kon*, have been credited with many phytotherapeutic successes in Japanese and Chinese folk medicine.[5,6] Today's biological interest in resveratrol was stimulated by reports that polygonaceous plants rich in resveratrol have been extensively used in Japanese herbal folk medications for the treatment of inflammatory, fungal, bacterial, and lipid atherosclerosis ailments.[7] Thus the roots of *Polygonum cuspidatum* Sieb. et Zucc. (family Polygonaceae) and *Polygonum multiflorum* Thumb. (family Polygonaceae).[8,9] are potential natural sources of resveratrol and its derivatives. Other potential sources of resveratrol include *Pterolobium hexapetallum*, a nonedible legume;[10] heartwoods of *Cassia garrettiana* Caraib (family Leguminosae); a plant widely available in Peru known as *Cassia quinquangulata* Rich. (family Leguminosae);[11] cotyledons of groundnuts *Arachis hypogaea;*[12] *Eucalyptus globulus* Labill. (Myrtaceae); and *Bauhinia racemosa* Lamk.[13] The biosynthesis (formation from other constituents within the plant or fruit) of resveratrol in these natural sources is greatly increased in response to infection, wounding, and ultraviolet (UV) light irradiation, but not to natural sunlight.

Resveratrol has been reported to occur in two species of the well-known flowering plant "lilly," botanically known as *Veratrum grandiflorum* and *Veratrum formosanum*. The leaves of *Veratrum grandiflorum*,[14] and the roots and rhizomes of *Veratrum formosanum*, are able to biosynthesize resveratrol.[15] The latter has been used for many years in the Orient as a crude drug for the treatment of hypertension.

A major emphasis was placed on the presence of resveratrol in vines or grapes because of its function as a phytoalexin and its unique ability to protect against fungal infection.[16] The potential production of *trans*-resveratrol in response to UV radiation varies with grape maturity, state of ripening, and season. The synthesis of resveratrol is stimulated in vines and in peanuts under the conditions of external stimuli such as infection, UV light (but not natural sunlight), traumatic damage, or treatment with antifungal agents, detergents, heavy metals or chemicals.[17,18]

RESVERATROL IN GRAPES AND WINES

The consumption of grape products (e.g., berries, juice, puree, and wine) could be a way to incorporate a significant amount of resveratrol into the average diet. The presence of resveratrol has been confirmed in *Vitis vinifera* and *Vitis labrusca* grapes and in both white and red wines. As mentioned previously, resveratrol is also a natural constituent of bronze- and dark-skinned muscadine grapes (*Vitis rotundifolia*). Dark-skinned muscadine grapes have slightly higher concentrations of total resveratrol than most of the bronze-skinned counterparts. Muscadine wines compare favorably in resveratrol concentration with wines made from other species of grapes. But, unlike the seeds of *Vitis vinifera* and *Vitis labrusca*, the seeds of *Vitis rotundifolia* (muscadine grapes) have a high concentration of resveratrol.

The concentrations of *cis*- and *trans*-resveratrol isomers in

761 commercial red wines from fifteen countries and regions, without distinction as to grape varietal or vintage, were analyzed using a unique gas chromatography-mass spectrometry (GC-MS) analytical method.[1-3] In general, the lowest concentrations of *cis*- and *trans*-resveratrol were found in wines from areas that generally have warmer and drier climates, such as Italy, South America, South Africa, and California. The highest concentrations of *cis*-and *trans*-resveratrol were found in wines associated with harsher climates, such as Burgundy, Bordeaux, Switzerland, Oregon, and Canada. For example, Cabernet Sauvignon wines from California, Australia, and South America have much lower *trans*-resveratrol concentrations than those from Bordeaux and Ontario. The cooler and more humid conditions in the latter two regions may partly explain these differences in *trans*-resveratrol content.

Wines from Italy and the Iberian Peninsula, which are subject to warmer and drier conditions, tend to have low *trans*-resveratrol concentrations, yet the wines from the Rhône Valley, a relatively warm and dry place, have comparatively high *trans*-resveratrol concentrations. It is therefore probable that the differences between the wines from these three regions with similar climates are due to the intrinsic resveratrol-synthesizing capacity of the different cultivars employed. There is also the possibility that the nutrient supply of the soil and water plays a role in the levels of resveratrol in grapes from the different regions. Commercial red wines from Burgundy have the maximum amounts of *cis*- (11 millimols per liter) and *trans*-resveratrol (26 millimols per liter), while those from Spain and Portugal have the least.

Resveratrol glucosides are also important components of commercial wines.[4] Glucosides of *cis*- and *trans*-resveratrols are known as *cis*-polydatin (also known as *cis*-piceid) and *trans*-polydatin (also, known as *trans*-piceid). The highest values of total resveratrol glucosides were observed in red wines from Midi (18.9 millimols per liter), followed by Canada (15 millimols per liter), the Rhône Valley (14.6 millimols per liter), and Spain and Portugal (14.5 millimols per liter). A resveratrol glucosides content of greater than 12 millimols per liter was found in the wines from South America, Italy, and Central Europe.[4] An inverse relationship exists between resveratrol isomers and resveratrol glucosides, so that Burgundy wines have low polydatin and high resveratrol contents. Dr. Mattivi and his collaborators[5] have reported the resveratrol content for Cabernet Sauvignon wines of three vintages: The oldest vintage had the highest *trans*-resveratrol concentration, and the youngest one had the lowest. The concentration of *trans*-resveratrol has been found to remain very stable when wine samples have been stored in dark glass bottles, both at room temperature and at 4°C, and without exposure to direct sunlight.

THE CHEMISTRY AND BIOSYNTHESIS OF RESVERATROL

In 1976, Drs. Langcake and Pryce reported the presence of resveratrol and its derivatives in grapevine tissues.[1-3] It was discovered at that time that plants produced resveratrol when they were under attack by fungi, bacteria, or viruses. This led to the conclusion that resveratrol was a natural protectant to plants under times of stress, and also led to the beginning of studies to examine whether resveratrol could be beneficial to humans. Plant antibiotics such as resveratrol are known as phytoalexins. These compounds are the members of the plant kingdom classified as spermatophytes.

The chemical structure of resveratrol is important because from its structure chemists can determine some properties related to its benefit. Figure 1 shows the molecular structure of *cis*- and *trans*-resveratrol and some of their derivatives. The hexagons in the figure are called aromatic rings, and the OH groups are called hydroxyl groups. When aromatic rings and hydroxyl groups are together the chemical is called a phenol. Since there are more than one of these phenols present, the compounds are called polyphenols. Polyphenols are often associated with compounds that are antioxidants. This is because they can react with radicals to form a more stable molecule; one that is less toxic than the original radical. Figure 2 shows the way resveratrol and its derivatives are biosynthesized naturally in plants.

BIOAVAILABILITY OF RESVERATROL

Both the absorption and bioavailability of resveratrol have been extensively studied in animals and humans. Bioavailability is a measurement of how much of the medicinal substance actually gets into the blood via different modes of administration. For resveratrol, the mode of administration is oral. Moderate dosages of resveratrol induce significant pharmacological and therapeutic effects.

Bertelli and his collaborators[1] have evaluated the absorption, distribution, and excretion of natural *trans*- and *cis*-resveratrol after oral administration of red wine to rats. The first group of animals was given a daily oral dose of 4 milliliters of red wine containing 6.5 milligrams per liter of total resveratrol for fifteen days, while a second group of rats was fed a daily dose of 2 milliliters of red wine containing 6.5 milliliters per liter of total resveratrol for fifteen days. Total resveratrol concentrations were measured in plasma, urine, heart, liver, and kidney. Resveratrol was shown to be

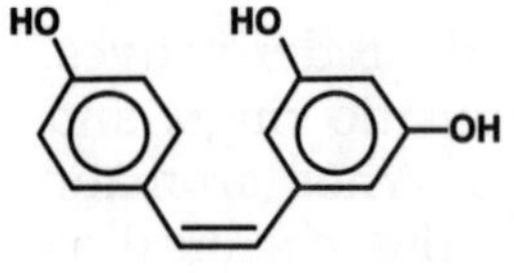

***cis*-resveratrol**

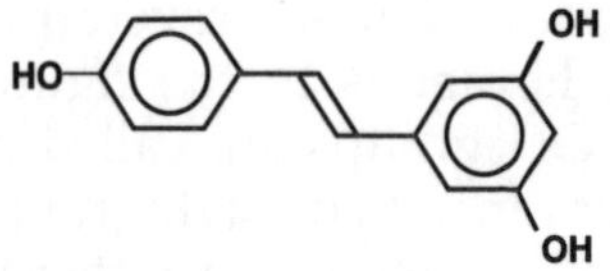

***trans*-resveratrol**

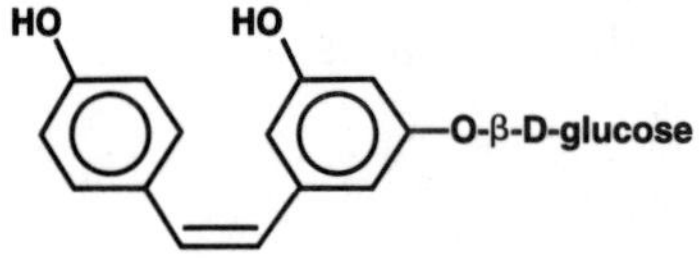

***cis*-resveratrol glucoside**

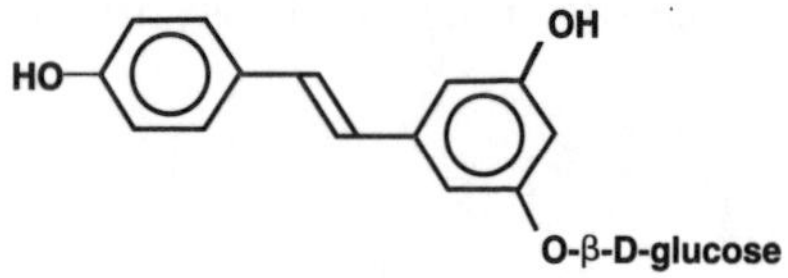

***trans*-resveratrol glucoside**

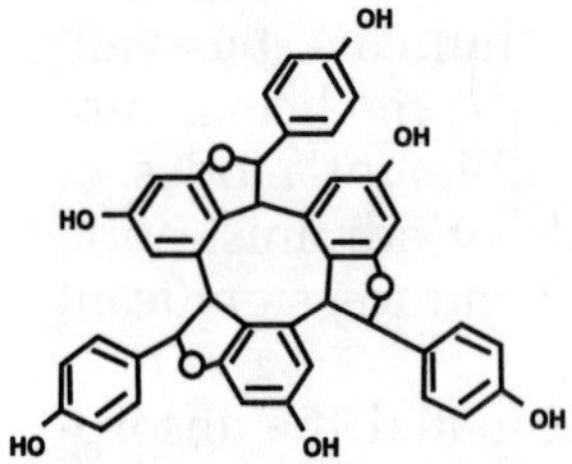

α-Viniferin

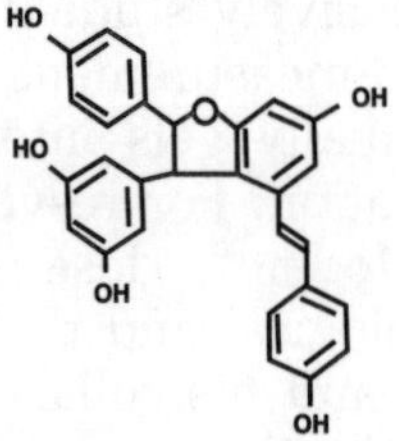

ε-Viniferin

Figure 1. Resveratrol and derivatives

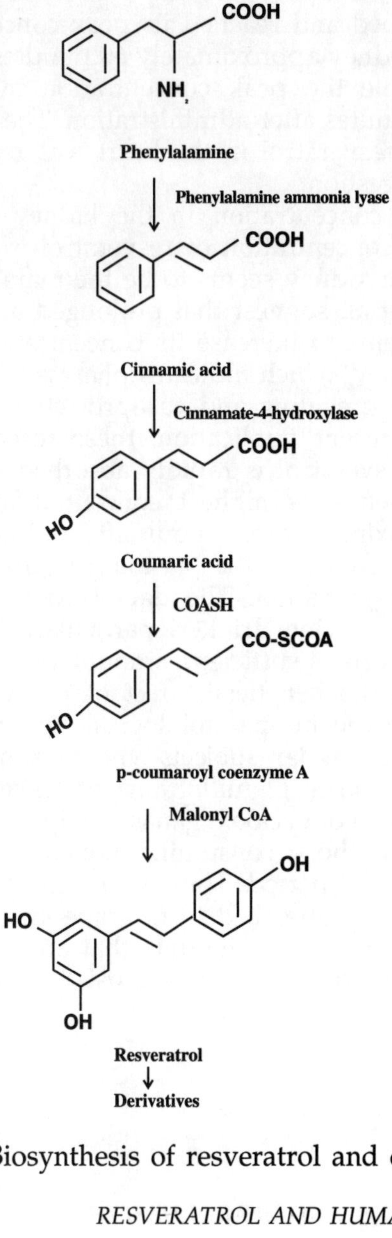

Figure 2. Biosynthesis of resveratrol and derivatives

quickly absorbed and reached its peak concentration in the plasma and kidney approximately 60 minutes after red wine ingestion, while the peak concentration in the liver was reached 30 minutes after administration. The maximum concentration of resveratrol in the heart was reached after 120 minutes of ingestion.

Resveratrol concentration in the kidney decreases with time. A high concentration of resveratrol is excreted in the urine; thus the kidney seems to be the main route of excretion. Bertelli et al. suggest that prolonged administration of resveratrol seems to increase its concentration in the heart, liver, and kidney, which indicates pharmacological activities such as anti-aggregating and vasoprotective action.

In a more recent publication, these researchers demonstrated that resveratrol is rapidly absorbed at the intestinal level and reaches its highest concentration in the blood plasma approximately one hour after administration. The concentrations found in the plasma are sufficient to invoke platelet anti-aggregation. The data lead to the conclusion that an average wine drinker, particularly over the long-term, can absorb a sufficient amount of resveratrol. This could explain the beneficial effect of red wine on human health as observed in epidemiological studies.[2]

Platelets from human subjects who consumed resveratrol-enriched grape juice (2 milligrams of resveratrol per day) had a lower ratio of cyclooxygenase to lipoxygenase product formation than those consuming nonenriched grape juice during the control period. The authors concluded that *trans*-resveratrol can be absorbed from grape juice in biologically active quantities and in amounts that are likely to cause a reduction in the risk of atherosclerosis.[3]

BIOLOGICAL EFFECTS OF RESVERATROL

In vitro and *in vivo* animal and human studies have shown that resveratrol possesses many biological attributes. These factors favor cardiovascular protection, neuroprotection,[1,2] antioxidative[1] and immunomodulatory activities, modulation of hepatic lipid synthesis, inhibition of platelet aggregation,[3] vasorelaxing effects, and inhibition of pro-atherogenic eicosanoids by human platelets and neutrophils.

Since resveratrol is a component of red wine (less than 1 to 13.4 milligrams resveratrol per liter), it has been postulated that resveratrol may be responsible for many of the health benefits attributed to red wine consumption. Resveratrol has been shown to act as an antimutagen by inhibiting the cellular events associated with tumor initiation, promotion, and progression. Resveratrol acts as a phytoestrogen and can serve as a natural replacement for estrogen during menopause. It has also been shown to decrease tumor growth *in vivo*. A recent study indicates that resveratrol directly stimulates cell proliferation and differentiation of osteoblasts, reduces the risk of osteoporosis, and increases bone formation. Other beneficial effects include increases in collagen synthesis and amelioration of depression. The following section is a summary of the biological effects reported for resveratrol.[1-6]

ANTIOXIDANT BENEFITS OF RESVERATROL

- Protects against free radical injury *in vivo*
- Inhibits hydroxyl and peroxyl radicals
- Increases plasma and LDL polyphenols
- Inhibits brain monoamine oxidase *in vivo*

Resveratrol reduced oxidative stress in cultured brain cells (PC12 cells) induced by the addition of Fe^{2+} and t-butyl hydroperoxide, and increased the antioxidant protective effects of vitamins C and E under these same conditions.[1]

Resveratrol also protected against free radical injury in cerebral ischemia. Ischemia refers to the obstruction of blood and oxygen flow through an organ, while restoration of blood and oxygen flow is termed reperfusion. Reperfusion induces more oxidative stress and damage to an organ than ischemia does.

In an ischemia-reperfusion rat brain model, resveratrol glycoside decreased levels of free radicals and lipid peroxidation (as demonstrated by a reduction in malondialdehyde production) and increased the antioxidant activities of antioxidant enzymes such as superoxide dismutase, catalase, and glutathione peroxidase. A concentration of 10 milligrams per kilogram body weight had the greatest effect.[2] Resveratrol increased plasma and LDL polyphenols and enhanced antioxidant activity as judged by decreased plasma peroxides. It also increased lag time and decreased LDL lipid peroxides and lipid peroxidation in the copper-catalyzed peroxidation of LDL conjugated dienes.[3]

Protykin, a natural extract of *trans*-resveratrol (20 percent) derived from the dried rhizome of *Polygonum cuspidatum*, scavenged both hydroxyl and peroxyl radicals *in vitro*, and provided significant cardioprotection *in vivo*. Supplementation of protykin to rats for three weeks dramatically improved postischemic left ventricular functions and aortic flow as compared to control animals. This was further supported by reduced myocardial (heart) infarct size, as measured by a computerized TTC staining method, and reduced malondialdehyde formation, a presumptive marker of oxidative stress. The researchers showed that protykin demonstrated dramatic cardioprotection, presumably by virtue of its potent free radical scavenging ability.[4]

Peroxidation of the LDL cholesterol from two healthy volunteers was inhibited by 81 percent and 70 percent upon the addition of 10 μmol per liter of *trans*-resveratrol (2.5 mg per liter). In contrast, 10 μmol per liter of α-tocopherol (natural vitamin E), which has been associated with a reduced risk of heart disease, had a much lower antioxidant potency than did resveratrol, and inhibited LDL cholesterol oxidation by only 40 percent and 19 percent.[5]

Inhibition of monoamine oxidase A was seen to be the prime factor responsible for the antioxidant activity of resveratrol. Monoamine oxidase is an enzyme found in most tissues, but especially in the liver and nervous system. It catalyzes the oxidation of a large variety of monoamines, including epinephrine, norepinephrine, and serotonin. Resveratrol and its derivatives induced a significant inhibitory effect on malonaldehyde generation—a marker of lipid peroxidation and oxidative tissue injury—during thrombin-induced platelet aggregation. Resveratrol also inhibited brain monoamine oxidase in rats (IC$_{50}$ of 2 μM), even though lacking the structural features of classic monoamine oxidase inhibitors. It is thought that inhibiting monoamine oxidase in the brain may be a way to treat depression.[6]

See pp. 66-67

RESVERATROL: A NATURAL PHYTOESTROGEN THAT INHIBITS THE GROWTH OF HUMAN BREAST CANCER CELLS

- Acts as an agonist for estrogen receptors
- Serves as a safe, natural replacement for estrogen during menopause
- Reduces the risk of osteoporosis and increases bone formation
- Ameliorates depression
- Increases collagen synthesis

The low incidence of breast, endometrial, ovarian, and prostate cancers has been demonstrated among vegetarians and Asians, who normally possess higher blood levels of phytoestrogens.[1-4] This epidemiological evidence supports the chemopreventive efficacy of phytoestrogens[1]. Phytoestrogens are naturally occuring plant-derived nonsteroidal compounds that are structurally or functionally similar to steroidal estrogens produced by the body, such as estradiol. Studies have demonstrated the health benefits of phytoestrogens, which address climacteric syndromes in women, including vasomotor symptoms and postmenopausal health risks, as well as exhibited anticarcinogenic properties.[1-3] Phytoestrogens provide protection against estrogen-dependent cancers, such as breast and prostate cancers, as well as promote bone health. Phytoestrogens inhibit angiogenesis, cell cycle progression, and aromatase enzyme inhibition. They also stimulate sex hormone–binding globulin synthesis, antioxidant properties, and digitalis-like activity.[3]

The main classes of phytoestrogens are isoflavonoids, phytoalexins, and coumestans. Asian populations, such as those of Japan, Taiwan, and Korea, are estimated to consume 20–150 milligrams per day of isoflavones, in the form of tofu and miso, with an average daily intake of 40 milligrams.[3] Red wine, which is high in the phytoalexin resveratrol, is known to be more estrogenic than beer or bourbon because of its resveratrol content. Beer and bourbon contain other phytoestrogens, but not resveratrol.

Enzymatic metabolic reactions, with conversions in the gastrointestinal tract, can be observed in females who have consumed red wine, which contains *trans*-resveratrol. These reactions produce compounds with structures similar to those in estrogens. The phytoestrogen metabolites are metabolized in the liver and are then expelled in the urine.[5]

Several authors have reported a decrease in hot flashes in Japanese women who had consumed phytoestrogens. Furthermore, dietary phytoestrogens prevent bone loss and fracture as well as osteoporosis.[6,7] Consumption of *trans*-resveratrol from red wine demonstrated beneficial effects in postmenopausal women by alleviating menopausal symptoms.[6,7]

It has been demonstrated that women who drink two glasses of red wine with a meal have a reduction in hot flashes, depression, and osteoporosis. Based on the reported levels of resveratrol found in red wine, a 750-milliliter bottle of quality red wine may contain as much as 500 μg of resveratrol. Thus, two glasses (400 milliliter) of red wine could provide approximately 265 μg of resveratrol. These levels of resveratrol may be sufficient to reduce estrogen-binding, which may in turn provide some beneficial effects in other areas, such as breast cancer.[6]

Phytoestrogens are known to bind and activate the estrogen receptor, but most phytoestrogens are less active than the endogenous estrogens. The natural phytoestrogen resveratrol exerts its dramatic antiestrogenic activity by preventing more potent endogenous estrogen from binding to the estrogen receptor.[1–3,5]

In a clinical trial, postmenopausal women randomized

to receive 100 μg per day of *trans*-resveratrol for six months (four glasses of red wine per day for six months) had increased bone mineral content and density.[8,9] Dr. Gehm hypothesized that, due to the structural similarity of the phenolic "A"-ring in both steroidal estrogens and in resveratrol, resveratrol might interact with the estrogen receptors.[10] He later showed that resveratrol competes with 17 β-estradiol to bind to the human estrogen receptor and helps menopausal women ameliorate estrogen-dependent cancer.

It is important to mention that menopause is not simply a condition of estrogen deficiency, but that it is a different estrogenic state altogether. After menopause, estrogen becomes estrone as a result of reduced estradiol secretion by the ovaries.[3] Following menopause, diethylstilbestrol (4,1'-dihydroxy-*trans*-α,β-diethylstilbene) and ethynylestradiol—synthetic hormones—are extensively used as replacement estrogen therapy. Resveratrol has a similar effect and benefit to diethylstilbesterol and estradiol.

Dr. Gehm demonstrated that during premenopause, 60 percent of estrogens come from estradiol secreted by the ovaries and 40 percent from estrone secreted via peripheral tissues by androstenedione conversion. After menopause, estrogen is secreted almost exclusively by the peripheral tissues. Estrogen levels can be increased by resveratrol supplementation, which enhances estrogen production. *Trans*-resveratrol stimulates low concentrations (3 to 10 μg) of estrogen secretion in the body, inhibits the binding of labeled estradiol to the estrogen receptor, and activates transcription of estrogen-responsive reporter genes that are transferred into human breast cancer cells.[10] Drs. Lu and Serrero of the University of Maryland School of Pharmacy have shown that resveratrol inhibits the growth of estrogen receptor-positive human breast cancer cells.[11] These scientists demonstrated that resveratrol antagonizes the breast cancer cell growth-stimulatory effect of estradiol in a dose-dependent fashion, both at the cellular level (cell-growth) and at the molecular level (gene activation).

Furthermore, resveratrol has a direct stimulatory effect on bone formation in cultured osteoblastic cells *in vitro*, and so may serve as a useful tool in the prevention of and therapy for osteoporosis. Alkaline phosphatase (ALP) activity is the most widely recognized biochemical marker for osteoblastic activity, and plays a role in bone mineralization. Resveratrol was seen to dose-dependently increase ALP activity and DNA synthesis in osteoblastic MC3T3-E1 cells. Thus, resveratrol stimulates the proliferation and differentiation of osteoblasts.

In addition, resveratrol accelerated prolyl hydroxylase activity, indicating that it increased collagen synthesis activity. These results suggest the stimulatory nature of resveratrol toward the function of osteoblastic cells. The stimulatory effects of resveratrol on ALP activity and DNA synthesis were clearly blocked by the presence of tamoxifen, an anti-estrogenic drug. The ability of resveratrol to increase bone formation is mediated through an estrogen-like action.[12]

Estrogens are essential for the development and function of female sex organs, as well as maintenance of bone strength, cardiovascular health, and brain function. With advancing age, women produce less estrogen and experience midlife changes. A broad spectrum of evidence suggests that phytoestrogen supplementation offers a potential alternative or complement to conventional hormone replacement therapy (HRT). Conventional HRT drugs, especially diethylstilbesterol, have been demonstrated to cause serious side effects including stroke, gallbladder disease, and certain types of cancer. Figure 3 represents the chemical structures of *trans*-resveratrol, diethylstilbesterol, and estradiol, showing similarity and affinity toward estrogen receptors. Studies have shown that *trans*-resveratrol enhances estrogen metabolism through the formation of a complex with estrogen receptors and can help women maintain normal estrogenic activity, reduce hot flashes, balance mood swings, maintain healthy bone density, promote cardiovascular health, and prevent the effects of premature aging.

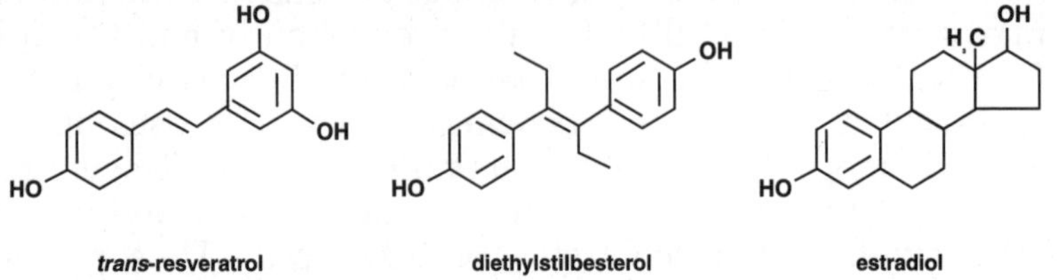

trans-resveratrol   diethylstilbesterol   estradiol

Figure 3. Chemical structures of *trans*-resveratrol, diethylstilbesterol, and estradiol

ANTIMUTAGENIC AND ANTICARCINOGENIC POTENTIAL OF RESVERATROL

- Stops the initiation, promotion, and progression of carcinogenesis
- Decreases tumor growth *in vivo*

Resveratrol has been demonstrated to inhibit the initiation, promotion, and progression stages of carcinogenesis. In January 1997, Dr. Jang and his collaborators[1] published a cutting-edge research results in *Science*, considered the top-rated peer-reviewed journal. Their work showed that resveratrol functions as a potent antimutagen. Its beneficial effects included the induction of Phase II drug-metabolizing enzymes (anti-initiation activity), inhibition of cyclooxygenase and hydroperoxidase functions (antipromotion activity), and the induction of human promyelocytic-leukemic cell differentiation (antiprogression activity). Thus, resveratrol inhibits three prime stages of carcinogenesis: initiation, promotion, and progression. In addition, resveratrol inhibited the development of preneoplastic lesions in carcinogen-treated mouse mammary glands *in vitro*, and inhibited tumorigenesis in a mouse skin-cancer model.

Resveratrol inhibited cancer initiation by reducing *in vitro* free radical formation when human leukemia cells were treated with TPA effective dose [ED_{50}] of 27 μM,[2] inhibiting the mutagenic response when *Salmonella typhimurium* cells were treated with a noxious polycyclic aromatic hydrocarbon DMBA (ED_{50} of 4 μM),[3] and inducing quinone reductase activity in cultured mouse hepatoma cells (ED_{50} of 21 μM).[4] This last observation is highly significant because Stage II enzymes such as quinone reductase are capable of detoxifying carcinogens.[5]

Resveratrol-inhibited cancer promotion in mice by inhibiting cyclooxygenase activity of COX-1 (ED_{50} of 15 μM) and hydroperoxidase activity of COX-1 and COX-2 (ED_{50} of 3.7 μM and 85 μM, respectively); and reducing pedal edema both in the acute (3 to 7 hours) and chronic (24 to 144 hours) phases.[1] Cyclooxygenase activity inhibition is relevant to cancer chemoprevention because it catalyzes the conversion of arachidonic acid to pro-inflammatory substances, which can stimulate tumor cell growth and suppress immune surveillance.[6] Cyclooxygenase can also activate carcinogens to forms that damage cellular material.[7]

Considerable evidence has accumulated suggesting that COX-2 is important in tumorigenesis and that targeted inhibition of COX-2 may be an innovative approach to preventing cancer and treating inflammation. Treatment of human mammary epithelial cells with phorbol ester (PMA)– mediated induction of COX-2 induces a marked increase in production of prostaglandin E_2. The enhanced synthesis of prostaglandins can favor the growth of malignant cells by increasing cell proliferation. Resveratrol suppresses PMA-mediated increases in COX-2 mRNA and protein. Additionally, nuclear runoffs revealed increased rates of COX-2 transcription after treatment with PMA, an effect that also was inhibited by resveratrol. In this way, resveratrol can serve as a potential natural product to prevent cancer by targeted inhibition of COX-2.[8]

Resveratrol delayed the onset of cancer progression by inducing expression of nitroblue tetrazolium reduction activity, a marker of granulocyte formation (ED_{50} of 11 μM), and nonspecific acid esterase activity, a marker of macrophage formation (ED_{50} of 19 μM); and inhibiting incorporation of [^{3}H]thymidine, a marker of terminal differentiation to a nonproliferative phenotype.[1]

Resveratrol demonstrated cancer chemoprotective activity *in vitro* by inhibiting development of DMBA (2,7-dimethylbenz[a]anthracene) induced preneoplastic lesions in cultured mice mammary glands (ED_{50} of 3.1 μM); and *in vivo* by reducing 12-O-tetradecanoylphorbol-13-acetate (TPA) induced tumor initiation and promotion in mice given 1, 5, 10 or 25 μM of resveratrol together with TPA twice a week for eighteen weeks. This lowered the number of skin tumors per mouse by 68 percent, 81 percent, 76 percent, and 98 percent, respectively, and reduced the percentage of mice with tumors by 50 percent, 63 percent, 63 percent, and 88 percent, respectively.[1]

Resveratrol was found to possess chemopreventive activity by inhibiting ribonucleotide reductase[9] and cyclooxygenase-2[8] and by inhibiting cellular events associated with cell proliferation and tumor initiation, promotion, and progression.[1,10]

Ribonucleotide reductase is a protein enzyme complex that catalyzes the reduction of ribonucleotides into the deoxyribonucleotides required for DNA synthesis. Basically, this enzyme provides proliferating cells with the deoxynucleotides required for DNA synthesis. By inhibiting this enzyme, resveratrol exhibits antiproliferating activity and so inhibits cancer cell proliferation and differentiation.

Resveratrol has been shown to inhibit NADH:ubiquinone

oxidoreductase[11] and DNA polymerase.[12] Resveratrol also demonstrated strong cancer chemopreventive property by dramatically inhibiting human cytochrome P450 1A1 activity.[13] The ability of resveratrol to inhibit these key enzymes explains its antimutagenic, antiproliferative, and anticarcinogenic potential.

A very significant decrease (25 percent) in the tumor cell content resulted when rats inoculated with a fast-growing tumor (the Yoshida AH-130 ascites hepatoma) were given resveratrol *in vivo*. The researchers were able to show that resveratrol caused apoptosis (programmed cell death) in the tumor cell population, which resulted in a decreased cell number of cancer cells.[14]

Resveratrol was also found to induce apoptotic (programmed) cell death in human leukemic HL-60 cells and in T47D breast carcinoma cells at doses minimally toxic to normal peripheral blood lymphocytes. Resveratrol-induced apoptosis is mediated via caspase activation inhibitable by tetrapeptide caspase inhibitors. Furthermore, resveratrol enhances *CD95L* expression and induces *CD95*, signaling dependent cell death in both tumor cell lines. The chemopreventive activity of resveratrol could be explained by the induction of *CD95*-dependent apoptotic cell death in tumor cells, leading to the inhibition of tumor initiation and progression.[15]

Several recent communications have highlighted the role of the *CD95-CD95L* system in drug-induced or immune-mediated clearance of tumor cells, suggesting that the fate of antitumor therapy might be determined by the balance between *CD95* and *CD95L* expression on tumor cells and on immune cells. Once triggered, the *CD95* receptor can activate a series of intracellular events that culminate in the death cascade composed of intracellular caspases. These observations have led to the suggestion that *CD95-CD95L*–mediated signaling might be one critical event in drug-induced tumor cell death.[15]

Dr. Ragione and his colleagues[16] investigated the activity of resveratrol on proliferation and differentiation of the human promyelocitic HL-60 cells. A concentration as low as 30 μM causes a complete arrest of proliferation and a rapid induction of differentiation towards a myelo-monocytic phenotype. Resveratrol induces a complete and reversible cell cycle arrest at the S-phase checkpoint. These studies demonstrated that resveratrol is a potential candidate for the development of anticancer treatment as well as for inhibiting lymphocyte proliferation during immunosuppressive therapies.[16]

INHIBITION OF PROTEIN TYROSINE KINASE ACTIVITY BY RESVERATROL

• Inhibits tyrosine kinase, a promoter of diverse degenerative diseases

Protein tyrosine kinase regulates cell proliferation, cell differentiation, and signaling processes in cells of the immune system. Uncontrolled signaling from receptor tyrosine kinases and intracellular tyrosine kinases can lead to inflammatory responses and to diseases such as cancer, atherosclerosis, and psoriasis.[1] Both resveratrol and resveratrol glycoside inhibit protein tyrosine kinase activity. Resveratrol demonstrated greatest tyrosine kinase inhibition ability (IC_{50} of 220 to 264 μM), while resveratrol glycoside demonstrated some activity (IC_{50} of 512 to greater than 2048 μM).[2]

CARDIOPROTECTIVE PROPERTIES OF RESVERATROL

- Inhibits LDL oxidation and platelet aggregation
- Reduces serum cholesterol and triglyceride levels
- Induces vasorelaxing effects
- Inhibits tissue factor expression in vascular cells
- Reduces myocardial infarction and ischemia-reperfusion injury
- Stimulates endogenous adenosine release and protects against chronic ischemia

Resveratrol induces leukotriene production in human neutrophils by inhibiting 5-lipoxygenase and 15-lipoxygenase, enzymes involved in the metabolism of arachidonic acid to leukotrienes (IC_{50} of 22.4 and 8.7 µM, respectively). These effects are independent of resveratrol's free-radical scavenging ability, since other more powerful antioxidants did not have the same effect. Leukotrienes are powerful mediators of inflammatory reactions and are thought to be involved in the cellular processes that contribute to atherosclerosis.[1]

At a concentration of 10 µM, resveratrol reduced thromboxane A_2 production in human blood platelet cells by approximately 60 percent. Thromboxane A_2 is a powerful eicosanoid produced from arachidonic acid and is involved in the propagation of blood platelet aggregation. Neither quercetin nor any of the other wine phenolics or antioxidants tested had any effect at this concentration.[1]

Resveratrol inhibited adenosine diphosphate (ADP)- and thrombin-induced platelet aggregation of healthy human blood plasma in a dose-dependent manner (IC_{50} of 129.9 and 164.7 µmol per liter, respectively). The IC_{50} concentrations were rather high, but were still three orders of magnitude lower than that of ethanol, even though the antiplatelet activity of ethanol has been advanced as one of the mechanisms involved in protection against cardiovascular disease[1].

Resveratrol demonstrated an inhibitory effect on platelet aggregation due to its influence on arachidonate metabolism. Resveratrol lowered platelet aggregation of healthy human blood plasma by 50.3 percent at a concentration of 3.45 μg per liter. Red wine containing 1.2 milligrams per liter of natural trans-resveratrol and 3.6 grams per liter of polyphenols diluted 1,000-fold (final resveratrol concentration: 1.2 μg per liter) inhibited platelet aggregation by 41.9 percent. By adding resveratrol to wine up to a concentration of 1.2 μg per liter, inhibition was raised to 78.5 percent. These results suggest that the antiaggregating activity of resveratrol is related to its concentration in wine.[2]

One hundred μg per one milliliter trans-resveratrol also lowered serotonin release from "aspirinated" platelets activated by thrombin or cathepsin G. This suggests that trans-resveratrol does not primarily interfere with the formation of prostaglandins and thromboxane in platelets, and that its inhibitory effect may be added to that of aspirin.[3]

In rats fed a high cholesterol diet, resveratrol inhibited cholesterol and triglyceride liver deposition, lowered serum triglyceride and low-density lipoprotein (LDL) cholesterol levels, reduced the atherogenic index (total cholesterol: high-density lipoprotein (HDL) cholesterol), and decreased the rate of hepatic triglyceride synthesis from [^{14}C]-palmitate.[4]

Resveratrol promoted both direct and indirect vasorelaxing effects on arterial vessels of rats by nitric oxide-mediated and non-nitric oxide-mediated mechanisms. At a concentration of 3×10^{-5}M, resveratrol caused vasorelaxation that was reversed by a 1×10^{-6}M concentration of nitric oxide synthetase inhibitor. At a higher concentration of 6×10^{-5}M, resveratrol induced vasorelaxation that could not be reversed by nitric oxide synthetase inhibitor. This indicates that resveratrol acts directly on vascular smooth muscle cells.[5]

Peroxidation of LDL cholesterol obtained from two

healthy volunteers by 81 percent and 70 percent was inhibited upon the addition of 10 μmol per liter of resveratrol. By contrast, 10 μmol per liter of alpha-tocopherol (natural vitamin E)—which has been associated with a reduced risk of heart disease—had a much lower antioxidant potency than resveratrol, and inhibited LDL cholesterol oxidation by only 40 percent and 19 percent.[6]

Resveratrol increased plasma and LDL polyphenols and enhanced antioxidant activity as judged by decreased plasma total peroxides, increased lag time, and decreased LDL lipid peroxides and lipid peroxidation in the copper-catalyzed peroxidation of LDL conjugated dienes.[7]

Protykin, a natural extract of trans-resveratrol (20 percent) derived from the dried rhizome of Polygonum cuspidatum, demonstrated excellent in vitro peroxyl radical [generated by 2,2'-azobis(2-amidinopropane) dihydrochloride] and hydroxyl radical (in a 7-OH-coumarin-3-carboxylic acid model) scavenging abilities; and provided significant cardioprotection in vivo. Myocardial protection of protykin was assessed in vivo to determine whether protykin could preserve the heart during ischemic arrest. In an in vivo ischemia-reperfusion model, three weeks of protykin supplementation to rats significantly improved postischemic left ventricular functions [dp, dp/dt_{max}] and aortic flow. It also reduced myocardial infarction (determined by TTC staining) and reduced malondialdehyde formation (a presumptive marker of oxidative stress) in the coronary effluent. Thus the researchers demonstrated that protykin offers dramatic cardioprotection, presumably by virtue of its potent free radical scavenging ability.[8]

Polyphenolic compounds are known to possess antioxidant, anti-atherogenic, antithrombotic, and platelet anti-aggregating activities. Very recently they have been shown to stimulate the release of adenosine, an endogenous nucleoside. Adenosine is considered to be one of the mediators—perhaps the only mediator—of the most important spontaneous organic protection against chronic ischemia, a phenomenon known as "ischemic preconditioning." Following oral administration of a single dose of resveratrol (1.5 milligrams per kilogram of body weight) to ten healthy human volunteers, plasma adenosine levels increased progressively and reached a peak 30 minutes after ingestion and then successfully decreased to the starting values at 120 minutes.[9]

ANTI-INFLAMMATORY AND IMMUNE-ENHANCING PROPERTIES OF RESVERATROL

- Reduces inflammation
- Enhances immune functions

Resveratrol reduced inflammatory response in rat peritoneal leukocytes by inhibiting enzymes involved in arachidonic acid metabolism. These included the 5-lipoxygenase pathway evaluated by the rate of 5-HETE production (IC_{50} of 2.72 µM), and the cyclooxygenase pathway evaluated by HHT and thromboxane B_2 production (IC_{50} of 0.68 and 0.81 µM, respectively).[1]

Leukotrienes are powerful mediators of inflammatory reactions and are thought to be involved in the cellular processes that contribute to atherosclerosis. Resveratrol reduced leukotriene production in human neutrophils by inhibiting 5-lipoxygenase and 15-lipoxygenase, the enzymes involved in the metabolism of arachidonic acid to leukotrienes (IC_{50} of 22.4 and 8.7 µM, respectively).[2] These effects were independent of resveratrol's free radical–scavenging ability, since other more powerful antioxidants did not have the same effect.

Resveratrol was demonstrated to increase the levels of cyclic adenosine monophosphate (cAMP) in human polymorphonuclear leukocytes. These are involved in a variety of inflammatory and immunological processes, such as release of histamine, leukotrienes, and lysosomal enzymes from the lungs and leukocytes.[3]

Currently considered as biomarkers of inflammation are intracellular cell adhesion molecules (ICAM-1), vascular cell adhesion molecules (VCAM-1), E-Selectin, and P-Selectin. Many pathological conditions—such as inflammation and acute or chronic rejection—are found to be characterized by enhanced adhesion of leukocytes to endothelium.[4, 5]

The ability of resveratrol to modify endothelial adhesion of neutrophils and monocytes was investigated by Dr. Ferrero and her collaborators. Resveratrol inhibited the expression of adhesion molecules ICAM-1 and VCAM-1 by tumor necrosis factor α (TNF-α) stimulated human umbilical vein endothelial cells and by lipopolysaccharide-stimulated human saphenous vein endothelial cells (HSVEC). In addition, resveratrol induced a significant inhibition in the adhesion of U937 monocytoid cells to lipopolysaccharide-stimulated HSVEC.[4,5] Modification of such adhesion by resveratrol may support its use as an immunomodulating agent, as well as its potential role as an anti-inflammatory or antirejecting compound.

The cellular transcription factor, NF-$\kappa\beta$ (nuclear factor–kappa beta), mediates immune and inflammatory responses and regulates a diverse group of genes involved in cell proliferation, oncogenesis, and apoptosis. The activation of these signal transduction pathways is regulated by protein tyrosine kinases, and the pathways have an important role in the regulation of transcription factors. More importantly, NF-$\kappa\beta$ is under the control of protein tyrosine kinases. Considerable evidence indicates that, after cellular stimulation, NF-$\kappa\beta$ translocation as well as NF-$\kappa\beta$ dependent gene expression can be suppressed by protein tyrosine kinase inhibitors. Resveratrol has been shown to inhibit cellular events associated with tumorigenesis and inflammatory response. Resveratrol treatment was also shown to block lipopolysaccharide-induced activation of NF-κβ in a dose-dependent manner. Furthermore, resveratrol was shown to regulate NF-κβ at the level of nuclear translocation.[6]

RESVERATROL AND NEUROPROTECTION

- Protects against dementia
- Reduces oxidative stress in brain cells
- Protects against free radical injury in cerebral ischemia
- Protects against depression

Alcohol has been shown to be noxious to the brain and peripheral nervous system. Excessive consumption of alcohol can lead to severe and complete derangement of the nervous system, which is correctly termed "alcoholic dementia."

In a recent epidemiological study performed in the Bordeaux region by Orgogozo et al., an inverse relationship was found between red wine intake and the occurrence of dementia in the elderly.[1,2] For women, two or three glasses of red wine a day, and for men, three to four glasses of red wine a day, gave the maximum protection from or at least a delay in the onset of dementia. However, increased wine intake led to a decrease in prevention. Thus, it is the nonalcoholic constituents of red wine that have demonstrated a broad spectrum of pharmacological, medicinal, and therapeutic neuroprotective properties.

Resveratrol is the most active and efficacious of the nonalcoholic constituents of wine. Studies have shown that resveratrol reduces oxidative stress in cultured brain cells.[3] Furthermore, resveratrol induced phosphorylation of the mitogen-activated protein (MAP) kinase family members—extracellular regulated kinase 1 (ERK1) and 2 (ERK2)—in human neuroblastoma SH-SY5Y cells *in vitro*.

In particular, phosphorylation of ERK2 has been related to the synaptic changes at the basis of memory and learning processes. Phosphorylation of ERK1 and ERK2 occurs with a very low concentration of resveratrol (1 pM) and increases to a concentration of up to 1 μM. This reaction decreases at higher concentrations and is even inhibited with respect to the control values of untreated culture at 50 and 100 μM concentrations. These data, in conjunction with the epidemiological studies, suggest that moderate red wine intake—especially resveratrol intake—may have a positive effect on brain cells and also protect against dementia.[4]

Resveratrol also showed significant protection against free radical injury in cerebral ischemia. In an ischemia-reperfusion rat brain model, resveratrol glycoside lowered levels of free radicals and lipid peroxidation, and increased the antioxidant activities of antioxidant enzymes such as superoxide dismutase, catalase, and glutathione peroxidase. A concentration of 10 milligrams per kilograms had the greatest effect.[5]

Resveratrol inhibited brain monoamine oxidase in rats (IC_{50} of 2 μM) and demonstrated itself as a potent monoamine oxidase inhibitor. Monoamine oxidase, an enzyme found in most tissues (especially in the liver and the nervous system) catalyzes the oxidation of a large variety of monoamines, including epinephrine, norepinephrine, and serotonin. Inhibition of monoamine oxidase in the brain may serve as a potential way for resveratrol to be used in treating depression.[6]

MECHANISM OF ACTION OF RESVERATROL

The previous chapters have illustrated the diverse protective abilities of the novel phytopharmaceutical known as resveratrol against a broad spectrum of degenerative diseases and dysfunctions. The following are major mechanistic pathways of cytoprotection by this novel phytoalexin.

Resveratrol:

- inhibits hydroxyl and peroxyl radicals
- induces Phase II–drug-metabolizing enzymes and potentiates cancer anti-initiation activity
- mediates anti-inflammatory effects and inhibits cyclooxygenase (COX) and hydroperoxidase functions
- induces cancer antipromotion activity and potentiates cancer antiprogression activity
- induces human promyelocytic leukemia cell differentiation
- induces carcinogen detoxification by inducing quaninone reductase activity
- inhibits ribonucleotide reductase, cyclooxygenase, cytochrome P450 1A1, DNA polymerase, and NADH:ubiquinone oxireductase enzyme activities. This ability to inhibit these key enzymes explains resveratrol's antimutagenic, antiproliferative, and anticarcinogenic potential.
- regulates nuclear transcription factor, NF-$\kappa\beta$, at the level of nuclear translocation
- inhibits brain monoamine oxidase *in vivo*
- enhances collagen synthesis
- functions as a novel phytoestrogen
- inhibits the expression of adhesion molecules ICAM-1 and VCAM-1.

HUMAN CLINICAL STUDIES ON RESVERATROL

As an antioxidant,[1,2] *trans*-resveratrol has health benefits associated with moderate wine consumption. The results of this study may be quite important in determining the relationship between wine and health.[3] Based on the reported levels of resveratrol found in red wine, a 750 milliliter bottle of red wine may contain as much as 500 μg of *trans*-resveratrol. Two glasses (400 milliliter) of this beverage could then provide approximately 265 μg of *trans*-resveratrol. These levels of *trans*-resveratrol may be sufficient to reduce estrogen binding, which may in turn provide beneficial effects in areas such as breast cancer. Resveratrol was shown to produce estrogenic effects in postmenopausal women, reducing hot flashes and alleviating menopausal symptoms. Postmenopausal women randomized to receive 100 μg per day of *trans*-resveratrol (equivalent to four glasses of red wine a day) for six months demonstrated increased bone mineral content and density.[4,5]

Oral administration of a single dose of resveratrol (1.5 milligrams per kilogram body weight) to ten healthy human volunteers stimulated the release of plasma adenosine (an endogenous nucleoside).[6] Adenosine levels increased progressively and reached a peak 30 minutes after ingestion and successfully decreased to the starting values at 120 minutes. Adenosine is considered to be one of the mediators of the most important spontaneous organic protection against chronic ischemia ("ischemic preconditioning"). This study demonstrates the protective ability of resveratrol against chronic ischemia.

Resveratrol lowered platelet aggregation of healthy human

blood plasma by 50.3 percent at a concentration of approximately 3.5 milligrams per liter. Red wine containing 1.2 milligrams per liter of natural *trans*-resveratrol and 3.6 grams per liter of polyphenols diluted 1,000-fold (final resveratrol concentration: 1.2 milligrams per liter) inhibited platelet aggregation by 42 percent. By adding resveratrol to wine up to a concentration of 1.2 milligrams per liter, inhibition was raised to 78.5 percent[7]. These results suggest that the anti-aggregating activity of resveratrol is related to its concentration in wine. Resveratrol also inhibited ADP- and thrombin-induced platelet aggregation of healthy human blood plasma in a dose-dependent manner (IC_{50} of 129.9 and 164.7 µmol per liter, respectively). The IC_{50} concentrations were rather high, but were three orders of magnitude lower than that of ethanol, although the antiplatelet activity of ethanol has been advanced as one of the mechanisms involved in its protective effects against cardiovascular disease.[8]

SAFETY OF RESVERATROL

The LD_{50} of polydatin in mice (a lethal dose from which 50 percent of the animals die) was 1,000 milligrams per kilograms, demonstrating the relative safety of this product. *In vitro* experiments were conducted to determine the lactate dehydrogenase release from leukocytes as a marker of cell membrane injury following incubation with different concentrations of resveratrol. Concentrations of 5×10^{-7} to 10^{-3} M did not cause release of more than 7 percent of lactate dehydrogenase from leukocytes, suggesting that it does not induce cell damage at these concentrations.

RECOMMENDED DOSES AND AVAILABILITY OF RESVERATROL

Resveratrol is a relatively new nutritional supplement demonstrating a broad spectrum of medicinal properties against cancer, osteoporosis, acute and chronic phases of inflammation, cardiovascular dysfunctions, and depression. It is a phytoestrogen. Further human clinical studies need to be conducted to determine more about its absorption, distribution, bioavailability, mechanism of action, dosage, and efficacy. Generally, one glass of red wine contains an average of approximately 650 micrograms of resveratrol, while a handful of peanuts contains approximately 75 micrograms of resveratrol.

The recommended adult daily dosage is 2 to 2.5 milligrams of *trans*-resveratrol. These recommendations are based, in part, on red wine content of resveratrol (less than 1 to 13.4 milligrams per liter), published human clinical dosage of resveratrol (2 milligrams per day), human-equivalency dose (HED) calculations of animal data (1.2 to 102 milligrams per effective dose), and commercially available resveratrol products (less than 1 to 10 milligrams per tablet or capsule).

Various companies make resveratrol. Natrol Inc. (Chatsworth, California) sells 10-milligram *trans*-resveratrol capsules in thirty- and sixty-capsule units, and this product is naturally extracted from *Polygonum cuspidatum* roots, which contain 20 percent *trans*-resveratrol, 24 percent total resveratrol, and 10 percent emodin. This resveratrol ingredient is commercially known as Protykin and is manufactured by InterHealth (Benicia, California), and recently published university studies have demonstrated that this product can provide dramatic cardioprotection in rats. InterHealth has recently introduced in the market another 50 percent extract of *trans*-resveratrol and 2 percent emodin from *Polygonum cuspidatum*. Source Naturals (Scotts Valley, California) also markets resveratrol antioxidant tablets containing 10 milligrams *trans*-resveratrol and other antioxidants. Nutraceuticals World, HSR Health Supplement Retailer, and Natural Products Industry Insider have listed a significant number of companies manufacturing resveratrol finished products. The list includes Reliance Vitamin, GCI Nutrients, Pharmline Inc., AIDP Inc., Ocean Spray, Phytochem, Stryka Botanicals, Maypro, American Ingredients, Triarco, Blue California Company, Tishcon Corporation, and others. Some of these companies also provide a combination of oligomeric proanthocyanidins and trace amount of *trans*-resveratrol.

Many of these products are available from a health food store or other outlets that specialize in natural product supplements and health products.

CONCLUSION

The novel phytopharmaceutical resveratrol, abundant in several plant species (such as grape skins, peanuts, and pine), is known to protect these plants against fungal infection and other diseases. Natural resveratrol has long been used as an integral component of an Oriental medicine known as *Ko-jo-kon*, claimed to have protective effects against arteriosclerosis and coronary heart disease. The roots of *Polygonum cuspidatum*, a novel natural source of resveratrol, have also been used to treat hyperlipidemia and arteriosclerosis, allergic diseases, and inflammatory responses. Recent studies have shown that resveratrol functions as a potent antioxidant, an immune-enhancer, an anti-inflammatory and anticancer agent, and is able to inhibit the cellular events associated with tumor initiation, promotion, and progression. Resveratrol inhibited cyclooxygenase activity of COX-1. Cyclooxygenase activity is relevant to cancer chemoprevention because this enzyme has the ability to catalyze the conversion of arachidonic acid to pro-inflammatory substances, which can stimulate tumor cell growth and suppress immune surveillance. Cyclooxygenase also activates carcinogens to promote cellular injury. Resveratrol inhibited cancer progression by inducing the expression of nitrobluetetrazolium reduction, a marker of granulocyte formation, and non-specific acid esterase activity, a marker of macrophage formation. Resveratrol also demonstrated potential chemopreventive activity by inhibiting several key enzymes responsible for cancer cell proliferation and differentiation including ribonucleotide reductase, cytochrome P450 1A1, protein tyrosine kinase, DNA polymerase, and NADH:ubiquinone oxidoreductase. *In vivo* oral administration of resveratrol caused a significant reduction in tumor growth and tumor cell count.

Resveratrol has demonstrated its ability to function as a neuroprotectant and to perform as a phytoestrogen, acting as a safe, natural replacement for estrogen during menopause, reducing the risk of osteoporosis, preventing depression, and increasesing bone formation and collagen synthesis. Resveratrol has exhibited a broad spectrum of cardioprotective properties, especially against chronic ischemia, myocardial ischemia-reperfusion injury, and myocardial infarction. Furthermore, resveratrol protects against LDL oxidation and platelet aggregation, and promotes vascular relaxation. Resveratrol has demonstrated its ability in neuroprotection as demonstrated by its action against dementia and depression, and its protection against free radical injury in cerebral ischemia.

Epidemiological data indicate that women on phytoestrogen-rich diets have less cardiovascular disease, breast and uterine cancer, and menopausal symptoms than those on Western diets. Preclinical and clinical studies have shown that phytoestrogens have lipid-lowering effects as well as the ability to inhibit low-density lipoprotein oxidation. *Trans*-resveratrol is a potent phytoestrogen and acts as an antioxidant, providing cellular protection against free radical attack, protecting the body against environmental pollutants, and retarding advancing age. Furthermore, *trans*-resveratrol has been shown to serve as a cardioprotectant and ameliorate postmenopausal symptoms including hot flashes, mood swings, vaginal itching and dryness, skin wrinkling, and decreasing bone strength, as well as prevent many of the problems diethylstilbesterol has been shown to cause.

The pharmacological, medicinal, and therapeutic properties of resveratrol strengthen the concept that regular supplementation of resveratrol may significantly contribute to disease prevention and the maintenance, protection, and promotion of good health.

Notes

Introduction

1. Pace-Asciak, C., Hahn, S., Diamandis E. P., Soleas, G., and Goldberg, D. M. "The Red Wine Phenolics trans-Resveratrol and Quercetin Block Human Platelet Aggregation and Eicosanoid Synthesis: Implications for Protection Against Coronary Heart Disease." Clin Chem Acta 235 (1995): 207–219.

2. Uenobe, F., Nakamura, S., and Miyazawa, M. "Antimutagenic Effect of Resveratrol against Trp-P-1." Mutat Res 373 (1997): 197–200.

3. Jang, M., Cai, L., Udeani, G. O., Slowing, K. V., Thomas, C. F., Beecher, C. W. W., Fong, H. H. S., Farnsworth, N. R., Kinghorn, A. D., Mehta, R. G., Moon, R. C., and Pezzuto J. M. "Cancer Chemopreventive Activity of Resveratrol, a Natural Product Derived from Grapes." Science 275 (1997): 218–220.

4. Frankel, E., Waterhouse, A. L., and Kinsella, J. E. "Inhibition of Human LDL Oxidation by Resveratrol. The Lancet 341 (1993): 1103–1104.

5. Fitzpatrick, D. F., Hirschfield, S. L., and Coffey, R. G. "Endothelium-Dependent Vasorelaxing Activity of Wine and Other Grape Products." American Journal of Physiology 265(2 pt 2) (1993): H774–H778.

The French Paradox and Coronary Heart Disease

1. St. Leger, A. S., Cochrane, A. L., and Moore, F. "Factors Associated with Cardiac Mortality in Developed Countries with Particular Reference to the Consumption of Wine." The Lancet 1 (1979): 1017–1020.

2. Criqui, M.H., and Ringel, B. L. "Does Diet or Alcohol Explain the French Paradox?" *The Lancet 344* (1994): 1719–1723.

3. Renaud, S. and de Lorgeril, M. "Wine, Alcohol, Platelets and the French Paradox for Coronary Heart Disease." *The Lancet 339* (1992): 1523–1526.

4. Gronbaek, M., Deis, A., Sorensen, T. I. A., Becker, U., Schnohr, P., and Jensen, G. "Mortality Associated with Moderate Intakes of Wine, Beer, or Spirits." *British Medical Journal 310* (1995): 1165–1169.

5. White, I. R. "The Cardioprotective Effects of Moderate Alcohol Consumption." *British Medical Journal 312* (1996): 1179–1180.

6. Frei, B. "Cardiovascular Disease and Nutrient Antioxidants: Role of Low-Density Lipoprotein Oxidation." *Crit Rev Food Sci Nutr 35 (1&2)* (1995): 83–98.

7. Marques-Vidal, P., Cambou, J. P., Nicaud, V., Luc, G., Evans, A., Arveiler, D., Bingham, A. and Cambien, F. "Cardiovascular Risk Factors and Alcohol Consumption in France and Northern Ireland." *Atherosclerosis 115* (1995): 225–232.

8. Woodward, M. and Tunstall-Pedoe, H. "Alcohol Consumption, Diet, Coronary Risk Factors, and Prevalent Coronary Heart Disease in Men and Women in the Scottish Heart Health Study." *J Epidemiol Common Health 49* (1995): 354–362.

9. Miller, G. J., Beckles, G. L. A., Maude, G. H., and Carson, D. C. "Alcohol Consumption: Protection Against Coronary Heart Disease and Risks to Health." *Intern J Epidemiol 19* (1990): 923–930.

10. Rimm, E. B., Giovannucci, E. L., Willet, W. C., Colditz, G. A., Ascherio, A., Rosner, B., and Stampfer, M. J. "Prospective Study of Alcohol Consumption and Risk of Coronary Disease in Men." *The Lancet 338* (1991): 464–486.

11. Rimm, E. B., Klatsky, A., Grobbee, D., and Stampfer, M. J. "Review of Moderate Alcohol Consumption and Reduced Risk of Coronary Heart Disease: Is the Effect Due to Beer, Wine, or Spirits?" *British Medical Journal 312* (1996): 731–736.

12. Anonymous. "Inhibition of LDL Oxidation by Phenolic Substances in Red Wine: A Clue to the French Paradox?" *Nutr Rev 51* (1993): 185–187.

Nutritional and Therapeutic Benefits of Wine

1. Goldberg, D. M. "Does Wine Work?" *Clin Chem 41* (1995): 14–16.

2. Goldberg, D. M., Hahn, S. E., and Parkes, J. G. "Beyond Alcohol: Beverage Consumption and Cardiovascular Mortality." *Clin Chem Acta* 237 (1995): 155–187.

3. Innes, G. "Cost-Effectiveness of Beer Versus Red Wine for the Prevention of Symptomatic Coronary Artery Disease." *Canadian Medical Association Journal 159* (1998): 1463–1466.

4. McDonald, J. B. "Not by Alcohol Alone." *Nutrition Today 14* (1979): 14–19.

5. German, J. B. "Nutritional Studies of Flavonoids in Wine," in: *Flavonoids in Health and Disease*, eds: C. A. Rice-Evans and L. Packer, Marcel Dekker Inc., New York, (1997) pp. 343–358.

6. Waterhouse, A. L., and Frankel, E. N. "Wine Antioxidants May Reduce Heart Disease and Cancer." Proceedings, OIV 73rd General Assembly, San Francisco, August 29–September 3, 1993, 11 Rue Roquepine, 75008 Paris, France, OIV, pp. 1–15.

7. Gehm, B. D., McAndrews, J. M., Chien, P. Y., and Jameson, L. "Resveratrol, a Polyphenolic Compound Found in Grapes and Wine is an Agonist for the Estrogen Receptor." *Proc. Natl Acad Sci USA 94* (1997): 14138–14143.

8. Kovac, V., Alonso, E., and Revilla, E. "The Effect of Adding Supplementary Quantities of Seeds during Fermentation on the Phenolic Composition of Wines." *Amer J Enol Vitic 46* (1995): 363–367.

9. Gorinstein, S., Zemser, M., Weisz, M., Haruenkit, R., and Trakhtenberg, S. "The Influence of Dry Matter of Different Alcoholic Beverages on Lipids, Proteins, and Antioxidant Activity in Serum of Rats." *Nutr Biochem 9* (1998): 131–135.

10. Whitehead, T. P., Robinson, D., Allaway, S., Syms, J., and Hale, A. "Effect of Red Wine Ingestion on the Antioxidant Capacity of Serum." *Clin Chem 41* (1995): 32–35.

11. Rifici, V. A., Stephan, E. M., Schneider, S. H., and Khachadurian, A. K. "Red Wine Inhibits the Cell-mediated Oxidation of LDL and HDL." *J Amer Coll Nutr 18* (1999): 137–143.

12. Roig, R., Cascon, E., Arola, L., Blade, C., and Salvado, M. J. "Moderate Red Wine Consumption Protects the Rat against Oxidation *in Vivo*." *Life Sci 64* (1999): 1517–1524.

13. Renaud, S. and Lorgeril, M. D. "Wine, Alcohol, Platelets, and the French Paradox for Coronary Heart Disease." *The Lancet 339* (1992): 1523–1526.

14. Morales, M., Alcantara, J., and Ros Barcelo, A. "Oxidation of

trans-Resveratrol by a Hypodermal Peroxidase Isozyme from Gamay Rouge Grape *(Vitis vinifera)* Berries." *Amer J Enol Vitic 48* (1997): 33–38.

15. Schwekendiek, A., Pfeffer, G., and Kindl, H. "Pine Stilbene Synthase cDNA, a Tool for Probing Environmental Stress." *FEBS Lett 301* (1992): 41–44.

16. Jeandet, P., Bessis, R., and Gautheron, B. "The Production of Resveratrol (3,5,4'-trihydroxystilbene) by Grape Berries in Different Developmental Stages." *Amer J Enol Vitic 42* (1991): 41–46.

17. Moreno-Manas, M., and Pleixats, R. "Dehydroacetic Acid Chemistry. A New Synthesis of Resveratrol, a Phytoalexin of *Vitis vinifera.*" *An Quim 81* (1985): 157–161.

18. Holmgren, E. "Why Wine Can Be Part of a Healthy Diet and Lifestyle." *ASEV Online,* June 24, 1996.

19. Holmgren, E. "Wine Better Than Other Alcoholic Drinks . . . for People and Rabbits." *Wine Trader,* 1996.

20. Waterhouse, A. L. "Wine and Heart Disease." *Chemistry and Industry* (May 1, 1995): 338–341.

21. Holmgren, E. "Wine Antioxidants and Health: In Search of Answers," *Wine Trader (1996).*

22. Jibrin, J. "Salute: New Reasons to Drink to Your Health." *Longevity* (February 1993): 56–58.

23. Suadicani, P., Hein, H. O., and Gyntelberg, F. "Strong Mediators of Social Inequalities in Risk of Ischaemic Heart Disease: A Six-year Follow-up in the Copenhagen Male Study." *International Journal of Epidemiology 26* (1997): 516–522.

24. Bonneaux, L., Looman, C. W., Barendregt, J. J., and Van der Maas, P. J. "Regression Analysis of Recent Changes in Cardiovascular Morbidity in The Netherlands." *British Medical Journal 314* (1997): 789–792.

Natural Sources of Resveratrol

1. Langcake, P., and Pryce, R. J. "The Production of Resveratrol by *Vitis vinifera* and Other Members of the *Vitaceae* as a Response to Infection and Injury." *Physiol Plant Pathol 9* (1976): 77–86.

2. Roggero, J. P., and Garcia-Parrilla, C. "Effects of Ultraviolet Irradiation on Resveratrol and Changes in Resversatrol and Various of its Derivatives in the Skins of Ripening Grapes." *Sci Aliments 15* (1995): 411–422.

3. Ector, B. J., Magee, J. B., Hegwood, C. P., Coign, M. J. "Resvera-

trol Concentration in Muscadine Berries, Juice, Pomace, Purees, Seeds and Wines." *Amer J Enol Vitic 47* (1996): 57–62.

4. Jeandet, P., Bessis, R., and Gautheron, B. "The Production of Resveratrol (3,5,4'-Trihydroxystilbene) by Grape Berries in Different Developmental Stages." *Amer J Enol Vitic 42* (1991): 41–46.

5. Nonomura, S., Kanagawa, H. and Makimoto, A. "Chemical Constituents of Polygonaceous Plants. I. Studies on the Components of Ko-jo-kon." *(Polygonum cuspidatum* Sieb. et Zucc.). *Yakugaku Zasshi 83* (1963): 988–990.

6. Kubo, M., Kimura, Y., Shin, H., Haneda, T., Tani, T., and Namba, K. "Studies on the Antifungal Substance of Crude Drug (II). On the Roots of *Polygonum cuspidatum* Sieb. et Zucc. (Polygonaceae)." *Shoyakugaku Zasshi 35* (1981): 58–61.

7. Nonomura, S., Kanagawa, H., and Makimoto, A. "Chemical Constituents of Polygonaceous Plants. I. Studies on the Components of Ko-jo-kon. *(Polygonum cuspidatum* Sieb et Zucc.)" *Yakugaku Zasshi 83* (1963): 988–990.

8. Kimura, Y., Okuda, H., and Arichi, S. "Effects of Stilbenes on Arachidonate Metabolism in Leukocytes." *Biochim Biophys Acta 834* (1985): 275–278.

9. Kimura, Y., Okuda, H., and Kubo, M. "Effects of Stilbenes Isolated from Medicinal Plants on Arachidonate Metabolism and Degranulation in Human Polymorphonuclear Leukocytes." *J Ethnopharmacology 45* (1995): 131–139.

10. Kumar, R. J., Jyostna, D., Krupadanam, G. L., and Srimannarayana, G. "Phenanthrene and Stilbenes from *Pterolobium hexapetallum." Phytochemistry 27* (1988): 3625–3626.

11. Jang, M., Cai, L., Udeani, G. O., Slowing, K. V., Thomas, C. F., Beecher, C. W. W., Fong, H. H. S., Farnsworth, N. R., Kinghorn, A. D., Mehta, R. G., Moon, R. C., and Pezzuto, J. M. "Cancer Chemopreventive Activity of Resveratrol, a Natural Product Derived from Grapes." *Science 275* (1997): 218–220.

12. Ingham, J. L. "3,5,4'-Trihydroxystilbene as a Phytoalexin from Groundnuts (*Arachis hypogaea*)" *Phytochemistry 15* (1976): 1791–1793.

13. Anjaneyulu, A. S. R., Raghava Reddy, A. V., Reddy, D. S. K., Ward, R. S., Adhikesavalu, D., and Cameron, T. S. "Pacherin: a New Dibenzo(2,3–6,7)oxepin Derivative from *Bauhinia racemosa* Lamk." *Tetrahedron 40* (1984): 4245–4252.

14. Hanawa, F., Tahara, S., and Mizutani, J. "Antifungal Stress

Compounds from *Veratrum grandiflorum* Leaves Treated with Cupric Chloride." *Phytochemistry 31* (1992): 3005–3007.

15. Chung, M. I., Teng, C. M., Cheng, K. L., Ko, F. N., and Lin, C. N. "An Antiplatelet Principle of *Veratrum formosanum*." *Planta Med 58* (1992): 274–276.

16. Goldberg, D. M., Yan, J., Ng, E., Diamandis, E. P., Karumanchiri, A., Soleas, G., and Waterhouse, A. L. "A Global Survey of *trans*-Resveratrol Concentrations in Commercial Wines." *Amer J Enol Vitic 46* (1995): 159–165.

17. Langcake, P., and Pryce, R. J. "The Production of Resveratrol and the Viniferins by Grapevines in Response to Ultraviolet Radiation." *Phytochemistry 16* (1976): 1193–1196.

18. Arora, M. K., and Strange, R. N. "Phytoalexin Accumulation in Groundnuts in Response to Wounding." *Plant Sci 78* (1991): 157–163.

Resveratrol in Grapes and Wines

1. Goldberg, D. M., Ng, E., Karumanchiri, A., Soleas, G., Yan, J., and Diamandis, E. P. "Regional Differences in Resveratrol Isomer Concentrations of Wines from Various Cultivars." *J Wine Res 7* (1996): 13–24.

2. Ector, B. J., Magee, J. B., Hegwood, C. P., and Coign, M. J. "Resveratrol Concentration in Muscadine Berries, Juice, Pomace, Purees, Seeds, and Wines." *Amer J Enol Vitic 47* (1996): 57–62.

3. Goldberg, D. M., Yan, J., Ng, E., Diamandis, E. P., Karumanchiri, A., Soleas, G., and Waterhouse, A. L. "A Global Survey of *trans*-Resveratrol Concentration in Commercial Wines." *Amer J Enol Vitic 46* (1996): 159–165.

4. Goldberg, D. M., Ng, E., Karumanchiri, A., Diamandis, E. P., and Soleas, G. "Resveratrol Glucosides are Important Components of Commercial Wines." *Amer J Enol Vitic 47* (1996): 415–420.

5. Mattivi, F. "Solid Phase Extraction of *trans*-Resveratrol from Wines and HPLC Analysis." *Z Lebensm Unters Forsch 196* (1993): 522–525.

The Chemistry and Biosynthesis of Resveratrol

1. Langcake, P., and Pryce, R. J. "The Production of Resveratrol by *Vitis vinifera* and Other Members of the *Viticeae* as a Response to Infection or Injury." *Physiol Plant Pathol 9* (1976): 77–86.

2. Langcake, P., and Pryce, R. J. "A New Class of Phytoalexins from Grapevines." *Experientia 33* (1977): 151–152.

3. Langcake, P., and Pryce, R. J. "The Production of Resveratrol and the Viniferins by Grapevines in Response to Ultraviolet Irradiation." *Phytochemistry 16* (1977): 1193–1196.

Bioavailability of Resveratrol

1. Bertelli, A. A. E., Giovannini, L., Stradi, R., Bertelli, A., and Tillement, J. P. "Plasma, Urine and Tissue Levels of *trans-* and *cis-*Resveratrol (3,5,4'-Trihydroxystilbene) after Short-term or Prolonged Administration of Red Wine to Rats." *Int J Tiss Reac 18* (1996): 67–71.

2. Bertelli, A., Bertelli, A. A. E., Gozzini, A., and Giovannini, L. "Plasma and Tissue Resveratrol Concentrations and Pharmacological Activity." *Drugs under Clinical and Experimental Research 24* (1998): 133–138.

3. Pace-Asciak, C., Rounova, O., Hahn, S. E., Diamandis, E. P., and Goldberg, D. M. "Wines and Grape Juices as Modulators of Platelet Aggregation in Healthy Human Subjects." *Clin Chim Acta 246* (1996): 163–182.

Biological Effects of Resveratrol

1. Chanvitayapongs, S., Draczynska-Lusiak, B., and Sun, A. Y. "Amelioration of Oxidative Stress by Antioxidants and Resveratrol in PC12 Cells." *Neuroreport 8* (1997): 1499–1502.

2. Leung, A., and Mo, Z. "Protective Effects of Polydatin, an Active Compound from *Polygonum cuspidatum*, on Cerebral Ischemia Damage in Rats." *Chin Pharm Bull 12* (1996): 128–129.

3. Nigdikar, S. V., Williams, N. R., Griffin, B. A., and Howard, A. N. "Consumption of Red Wine Polyphenols Reduces the Susceptibility of Low-Density Lipoproteins to Oxidation *in Vivo*." *Amer J Clin Nutr 68* (1998): 258–265.

4. Sato, M., Maulik, G., Bagchi, D., and Das, D. K. "Myocardial Protection by Protykin, a Novel Extract of *trans*-Resveratrol and Emodin." *Free Radical Research 32* (2000): 135–144.

5. Frankel, E., Waterhouse, A. L., and Kinsella, J. E. "Inhibition of Human LDL Oxidation by Resveratrol." *The Lancet 341* (1993): 1103–1104.

6. Han, Y. N., Ryu, S. Y., and Han, B. H. "Antioxidant Activity

of Resveratrol Closely Correlates with its Monoamine Oxidase-A Inhibitory Activity." *Arch Pharm Res 13* (1990): 132–135.

Antioxidant Benefits of Resveratrol

1. Chanvitayapongs, S., Draczynska-Lusiak. B., and Sun, A. Y. "Amelioration of Oxidative Stress by Antioxidants and Resveratrol in PC12 Cells.," *Neuroreport 8* (1997): 1499–1502.

2. Leung, A., and Mo, Z. "Protective Effects of Polydatin, an Active Compound from *Polygonum cuspidatum*, on Cerebral Ischemia Damage in Rats." *Chin Pharm Bulletin 12* (1996): 128–129.

3. Nigdikar, S. V., Williams, N. R., Griffin, B. A., and Howard, A. N. "Consumption of Red Wine Polyphenols Reduces the Susceptibility of Low-Density Lipoproteins to Oxidation *in Vivo*." *American Journal of Clinical Nutrition 68* (1998): 258–265.

4. Sato, M., Maulik, G., Bagchi, D., and Das, K. "Myocardial Protections by Protykin, a Novel Extract of *trans*-Resveratrol and Emodin." *Free Radical Research 32* (2000): 135–144.

5. Frankel, E., Waterhouse, A. L., and Kinsella, J. E. "Inhibition of Human LDL Oxidation by Resveratrol." *The Lancet 341* (1993): 1103–1104.

6. Han, Y. N., Ryu, S. Y., and Han, B. H. "Antioxidant Activity of Resveratrol Closely Correlates with its Monamine Oxidase-A Inhibitory Activity." *Arch Pharm Res 13* (1990): 132–135.

Resveratrol: A Natural Phytoestrogen That Inhibits the Growth of Human Breast Cancer Cells

1. Adlercreutz, H., Markkanen, H., and Watanabe, S. "Plasma Concentrations of Phytoestrogens in Japanese Men." *The Lancet 342* (1993): 1209–1210.

2. Stahl, S., Chun, T. Y., and Gray, W. G. "Phytoestrogens Act as Estrogen Agonists in an Estrogen-Responsive Pituitary Cell Line." *Toxicol Appl Pharmacol 152* (1998): 41–48.

3. Calabrese, G. "Nonalcoholic Compounds of Wine: The Phytoestrogen Resveratrol and Moderate Red Wine Consumption during Menopause." *Drugs Exptl Clin Res XXV* (1999): 111–114.

4. Lu, R., and Serrero, G. "Resveratrol, a Natural Product Derived from Grape, Exhibits Antiestrogenic Activity and Inhibits the Growth of Human Breast Cancer Cells." *J Cell Physiol 179* (1999): 297–304.

5. Adlercreutz, H., Fotsis, T., Heikkinen, R., Dwyer, J. T., Goldin,

B. R., Gorbach, S. L., Lawson, A. M., and Setchell, K. D. "Diet and Urinary Excretion of Lignans in Female Subjects." *Med Biol 59* (1981): 259–261.

6. Ashby, J., Tinwell, H., Pennie, W., Brooks, A. N., Lefevre, P. A., Beresford, N., and Sumpter, J. P. "Partial and Weak Oestrogenicity of the Red Wine Constituent Resveratrol: Consideration of Its Superagonist Activity in MCF-7 Cells and Its Suggested Cardiovascular Protective Effects." *J Appld Toxicol 19* (1999): 39–45.

7. Turner, R. T., Evans, G. L., Zhang, M., Maran, A., and Sibonga, J. D. "Is Resveratrol an Estrogen Agonist in Growing Rats?" *Endocrinology 140* (1999): 50–54.

8. Lock, M. "Ambiguities of Aging: Japanese Experience and Perceptions of Menopause." *Culture Med Psych 10* (1986): 23–46.

9. Anderson, J. J. B., and Garner, S. C. "Phytoestrogens and Bone." *Bailiers Clin Endocrinol Metab 12* (1998): 543–557.

10. Gehm, B. D., McAndrews, J. M., Chien, P. Y., and Jameson, J. L. "Resveratrol, a Polyphenolic Compound Found in Grapes and Wine, Is an Agonist for the Estrogen Receptor." *Proc Natl Acad Sci USA 94* (1997): 14138–14143.

11. Lu, R., and Serrero, G. "Resveratrol, a Natural Product Derived from Grape, Exhibits Antiestrogenic Activity and Inhibits the Growth of Human Breast Cancer Cells." *J Cell Physiol 179* (1999): 297–304.

12. Mizutani, K., Ikeda, K., Kawai, Y., and Yamori, Y. "Resveratrol Stimulates the Proliferation and Differentiation of Osteoblastic MC3T3 Cells. *Biochem Biophys Res Commun 253* (1998): 859–863.

Antimutagenic and Anticarcinogenic Potential of Resveratrol

1. Jang, M., Cai, L., Udeani, G. O., Slowing, K. V., Thomas, C. F., Beecher, C. W. W., Fong, H. H. S., Farnsworth, N. R., Kinghorn, A. D., Mehta, R. G., Moon, R. C., and Pezzuto, J. M. "Cancer Chemopreventive Activity of Resveratrol, a Natural Product Derived from Grapes. *Science 275* (1997): 218–220.

2. Sharma, S., Stutzman, J. D., Kelloff, G. J., and Steele, V. E. "Screening of Potential Chemoprotective Agents Using Biochemical Markers of Carcinogenesis." *Cancer Res 54* (1994): 5848–5855.

3. Shamon, L., Chen, C., Mehta, R. G., Steele, V., Moon, R. C., and Pezzuto, J. M. "A Correlative Approach for the Identification

of Antimutagens That Demonstrate Chemoprotective Activity." *Anticancer Res 14* (1994): 1775–1778.

4. Prochaska, H. and Santamaria, A. "Direct Measurement of NAD(P)H:quinone Reductase from Cells Cultured in Microliter Wells: A Screening Assay for Anticarcinogenic Enzyme Inducers." *Anal Biochem 169* (1988): 328–336.

5. Zhang, Y., Kensler, T. W., Cho, C. G., Posner, G. H., and Talalay, P. "Anticarcinogenic Activities of Sulphoraphane and Structurally Related Synthetic Norbornyl Isothiocyanates." *Proc Natl Acad Sci USA. 91* (1994): 3147–3150.

6. Plescia, O., Smith, A. H., and Grinwich, K. "Subversion of Immune System by Tumor Cells and Role of Prostaglandins." *Proc Natl Acad Sci USA 72* (1975): 1848–1851.

7. Wild, D., and Degan, G. "Prostaglandin H Synthase-dependent Mutagenic Activation of Heterocyclic Aromatic Amines of the IQ-type" *Carcinogenesis 8* (1987): 541–545.

8. Subbaramaiah, K., Chung, W. J., Michaluart, P., Telang, N., Tanabe, T., Inoue, H., Jang, M., Pezzuto, J. M., and Dannenberg, A. "Resveratrol Inhibits Cyclooxygenase-2 Transcription and Activity in Phorbol Ester-treated Human Mammary Epithelial Cells." *J Biol Chem 273* (1998): 21875–21882.

9. Fontecave, M., Lepoivre, M., Elleingand, E., Gerez, C., and Guittet, O. "Resveratrol, a Remarkable Inhibitor of Ribonucleotide Reductase." *FEBS Lett 421* (1998): 277–279.

10. Mgbonyebi, O. P., Russo, J., and Russo, I. H. "Antiproliferative Effect of Synthetic Resveratrol on Human Breast Epithelial Cells." *Int J Oncol 12* (1998): 865–869.

11. Fang, N., and Casida, J. E. "Anticancer Action of Cube Insecticide: Correlation for Rotenoid Constituents Between Inhibition of NADH:ubiquinone Oxidoreductase and Induced Ornithine Decarboxylase Activities." *Proc Natl Acad Sci USA 95* (1998): 3380–3384.

12. Sun, N. J., Woo, S. H., Cassady, J. M., and Snapka, R. M. "DNA Polymerase and Topoisomerase II Inhibitors from *Psoralea corylifolia.*" *J Nat Prod 61* (1998): 362–366.

13. Chun, Y. J., Kim, M. Y., and Guengereich, F. P. "Resveratrol Is a Selective Human Cytochrome P450 1A1 Inhibitor." *Biochem Biophys Res Commun 262* (1991): 20–24.

14. Carbo, N., Costelli, P., Baccino, F. M., Lopez-Sariano, F. J., and Argiles, J. M. "Resveratrol, a Natural Product Present in Wine,

Decreases Tumour Growth in a Rat Tumour Model." *Biochem Biophys Res Commun* 254 (1999): 739–743.

15. Clement, M. V., Hirpara, J. L., Chawdhury, S. H., and Pervaiz, S. "Chemopreventive Agent Resveratrol, a Natural Product Derived from Grapes, Triggers CD95 Signaling Dependent Apoptosis in Human Tumor Cells." *Blood 3* (1998): 996–1002.

16. Ragione, F. D., Cucciolla, V., Borriello, A., Pietra, V. D., Racioppi, L., Soldati, G., Manna, C., Galletti, P., and Zappia, V. "Resveratrol Arrests the Cell Division Cycle at S/G2 Phase Transition." *Biochem Biophys Res Commun* 250 (1998): 53–58.

Inhibition of Protein Tyrosine Kinase Activity by Resveratrol

1. Levitzki, A., and Gazit, A. "Tyrosine Kinase Inhibition: An Approach to Drug Development." *Science* 267 (1995): 1782–1788.

2. Jayatilake, G., Jayasuriya, H., Lee, E. S., Koonchanok, N. M., Geahlen, R. L., Ashendel, C. L., McLaughlin, J. L., and Chang, C. J. "Kinase Inhibitors from *Polygonum cuspidatum*." *J Nat Prod 56* (1993): 1805–1810.

Cardioprotective Properties of Resveratrol

1. Pace-Asciak, C., Hahn, S., Diamandis, E. P., Soleas, G., and Goldberg, D. M. "The Red Wine Phenolics *trans*-Resveratrol and Quercetin Block Human Platelet Aggregation and Eicosanoid Synthesis: Implications for Protection against Coronary Heart Disease." *Clin Chim Acta 235* (1995): 207–219.

2. Bertelli, A. A. E., Giovannini, L., Giannessi, D., Migliori, M., Bernini, W., Fregoni M., and Bertelli, A. "Antiplatelet Activity of Synthetic and Natural Resveratrol in Red Wine." *Int J Tiss Reac XVII* (1995): 1–33.

3. Rotondo, S., Evangelista, V., Manarini, S., de Gaetano, G., and Cerletti, C. "Red Wine, Aspirin and Platelet Function." *Thromb Haemost 76* (1996): 818–819.

4. Arichi, H., Kimura, Y., Okuda, H., Baba, K., Kozawa, M., and Arichi, S. "Effects of Stilbene Components of the Roots of *Polygonum cuspidatum* Sieb. et Zucc. On Lipid Metabolism." *Chem Pharm Bull 30* (1982): 1766–1770.

5. Chen, C., and Pace-Asciak, C. "Vasorelaxing Activity of Resveratrol and Quercetin in Isolated Rat Aorta." *Gen Pharmacol 27* (1996): 363–366.

6. Frankel, E., Waterhouse, A. L., and Kinsella, J. E. "Inhibition of Human LDL Oxidation by Resveratrol." *The Lancet 341* (1993): 1103–1104.

7. Nigdikar, S. V., Williams, N. R., Griffin, B. A., and Howard, A. N. "Consumption of Red Wine Polyphenols Reduces the Susceptibility of Low-density Lipoproteins to Oxidation *in vivo.*" *Amer J Clin Nutr 68* (1998): 258–265.

8. Sato, M., Maulik, G., Bagchi, D., and Das, D. K. "Myocardial Protection by Protykin, a Novel Extract of *trans*-Resveratrol and Emodin." *Free Radical Research 32* (2000): 135–144.

9. Blardi, P., De Lalla, A., Volpi, L., and Di Perri, T. "Stimulation of Endogenous Adenosine Release by Oral Administration of Quercetin and Resveratrol in Man." *Drugs Exptl Clin Res XXV* (1999): 105–110.

Anti-Inflammatory and Immune-Enhancing Properties of Resveratrol

1. Kimura, Y., Okuda, H. and Arichi, S. "Effects of Silbenes on Arachidonate Metabolism in Leukocytes." *Biochem Biophys Acta 834* (1985): 275–278.

2. Pace-Asciak, C., Hahn, S., Diamandis, E. P., Soleas, G., and Goldberg, D. M. "The Red Wine Phenolics *trans*-Resveratrol and Quercetin Block Human Platelet Aggregation and Eicosanoid Synthesis: Implications for Protection against Coronary Heart Disease." *Clin Chim Acta 235* (1995): 207–219.

3. Weissman, G. "Mechanisms of Lysosomal Enzymes Release from Leukocytes Exposed to Immune Complexes and Other Particles." *J Exp Med 134* (1971): 149s–165s.

4. Ferrero, M. E., Bertelli, A. A. E., Fulgenzi, A., Pellegatta, F., Corsi, M. M., Bonfrate, M., Ferrara, F., Caterina R. D., Giovannini, L., and Bertelli, A. "Activity *in vitro* of Resveratrol on Granulocyte and Monocyte Adhesion to Endothelium." *Amer J Clin Nutr 68* (1998): 1208–1214.

5. Ferrero, M. E., Bertelli, A. A. E., Pellegatta, F., Fulgenzi, A., Corsi, M. M., and Bertelli, A. A. "Phytoalexin Resveratrol (3,4',5-Trihydroxystilbene) Modulates Granulocyte and Monocyte Endothelial Adhesion." *Transplantation Proc 30* (1998): 4191–4193.

6. Holmes-McNary, M. Q., and Baldwin, A. S. Jr. "Nuclear Factor Kappa B (NF-κβ) Activation is Inhibited after Endotoxin Stimula-

tion by Resveratrol, a New Phytoalexin." *FASEB J 12* (1998): 2741, A472.

Resveratrol and Neuroprotection

1. Orgogozo, J. M., Dartigues, J. F., Lafont, S., Letenneur, L., Commenges, D., Salamon, R., Renaud, S., and Breteler, M. B. "Wine Consumption and Dementia in the Elderly: A Prospective Community Study in the Bordeaux Area." *Rev Neurology 153* (1997): 185–192.

2. Lemeshow, S., Letenneur, L., Dartigues, J. F., Lafont, S., Orgogozo, J. M., and Commenges, D. "Illustration of Analysis Taking into Account Complex Survey Considerations: The Association Between Wine Consumption and Dementia in the *PAQUID* Study. Personnes Ages Quid." *Amer J Epidemiol 148* (1998): 298–306.

3. Chanvitayapongs, S., Draczynska-Lusiak, B., and Sun, A. Y. "Amelioration of Oxidative Stress by Antioxidants and Resveratrol in PC12 Cells." *Neuroreport 8* (1997): 1499–1502.

4. Tredici, G., Miloco, M., Nicolini, G., Galbiati, S., Cavaletti, G., and Bertelli, A. "Resveratrol, MAP Kinases and Neuronal Cells: Might Wine Be a Neuroprotectant?" *Drugs Exptl Clin Res XXV* (1999): 99–103.

5. Leung, A., and Mo, Z. "Protective Effects of Polydatin, an Active Compound from *Polygonum cuspidatum*, on Cerebral Ischemia Damage in Rats." *Clin Pharm Bull 12* (1996): 128–129.

6. Han, Y. N., Ryu, S. Y., and Han, B. H. "Antioxidant Activity of Resveratrol Closely Correlates with its Monoamine Oxidase-A Inhibitory Activity." *Arch Pharm Res 13* (1990): 132–135.

Human Clinical Studies on Resveratrol

1. Bertelli, A. A. E., Giovannini, L., De Caterina, R., Bernini, W., Migliori, M., Fregoni, M., Bavaresco, L., and Bertelli, A. "Antiplatelet Activity of *cis*-Resveratrol." *Drugs Exptl Clin Res 22* (1996): 61–63.

2. Calabrese, G. "Nonalcoholic Compounds of Wine: The Phytoestrogen Resveratrol and Moderate Red Wine Consumption during Menopause." *Drugs Exptl Clin Res XXV* (1999): 111–114.

3. Ashby, J., Tinwell, H., Pennie, W., Brooks, A. N., Lefevre, P. A., Beresford, N., and Sumpter, J. P. "Partial and Weak Oestrogenicity of the Red Wine Constituent Resveratrol: Consideration of Its Su-

peragonist Activity in MCF-7 Cells and Its Suggested Cardiovascular Protective Effects." *J Appld Toxicol 19* (1999): 39–45.

4. Lock, M. "Ambiguities of Aging: Japanese Experience and Perceptions of Menopause." *Culture Med Psych 10* (1986): 23–46.

5. Anderson, J. J. B., and Garner, S. C. "Phytoestrogens and Bone." *Bailiers Clin Endocrinol Metab 12* (1998): 543–557.

6. Blardi, P., De Lalla, A., Volpi, L., and Di Perri, T. "Stimulation of Endogenous Adenosine Release by Oral Administration of Quercetin and Resveratrol in Man." *Drugs Exptl Clin Res XXV* (1999): 105–110.

7. Bertelli, A. A. E., Giovannini, L., Giannessi, D., Migliori, M., Bernini, W., Fergoni, M., and Bertelli, A. "Antiplatelet Activity of Synthetic and Natural Resveratrol in Red Wine." *Int J Tiss Reac XVII* (1995): 1–3.

8. Pace-Asciak, C., Hahn, S., Diamandis, E. P., Soleas, G., and Goldberg, D. M. "The Red Wine Phenolics *trans*-Resveratrol and Quercetin Block Human Platelet Aggregation and Eicosanoid Synthesis: Implications for Protection against Coronary Heart Disease." *Clin Chim Acta 235* (1995): 207–219.